CASES IN PATHOLOGY

A CLINICAL APPROACH FOR STUDENTS

CASES IN PATHOLOGY

A CLINICAL APPROACH FOR STUDENTS

Nancy Standler, M.D., Ph.D.

Department of Pathology
University of Pittsburgh
School of Medicine
Pittsburgh, Pennsylvania

Bernard Klionsky, M.D.

Professor and Vice Chairman
Department of Pathology
University of Pittsburgh
School of Medicine
Pittsburgh, Pennsylvania

Churchill Livingstone
New York, Edinburgh, London, Melbourne, Tokyo

Library of Congress Cataloging-in-Publication Data

Standler, Nancy.
    Cases in pathology : a clinical approach for students / Nancy
Standler, Bernard Klionsky.
       p. cm.
    Includes bibliographical references and index.
    ISBN 0-443-08759-8
    1. Pathology—Case studies. I. Klionsky, Bernard. II. Title.
    [DNLM: 1. Autopsy. 2. Pathology—case studies. QZ 4 S785c]
RB112.S73 1992
616.07—dc20
DNLM/DLC
for Library of Congress   91-29348
                                             CIP

© **Churchill Livingstone Inc. 1992**

Distributed in the United Kingdom by Churchill Livingstone, Robert Stevenson House, 1–3 Baxter's Place, Leith Walk, Edinburgh EH1 3AF, and by associated companies, branches, and representatives throughout the world.

Developmental Editor: *Margot Otway*
Copy Editor: *Elizabeth Bowman-Schulman*
Production Designer: *Charlie Lebeda*
Production Supervisor: *Christina Hippeli*
Cover design by Paul Moran

Printed in Hong Kong

First published in 1992   7 6 5 4 3 2 1

To the patients and their physicians
whose stories are told within these pages.

USING THIS BOOK

Cases in Pathology: A Clinical Approach for Students presents 37 cases from the files of the hospitals associated with the University of Pittsburgh School of Medicine. Each case contains a clinical history, a discussion of that history, information to put the case in a broader perspective, and photographs from the pathologic material associated with the case. The cases are designed as independent units and can be read in any order.

We have organized this material into chapters, each of which contains four or five cases pertaining to a particular organ system. The organization of the organ systems approximately follows that used by Robbin's *Pathologic Basis of Disease*. However, most cases present clinical information about several organ systems. Consequently, the reader is encouraged to consider cases in other chapters as well when reading about a particular organ system.

We have deliberately included cases that range from relatively simple to quite complex. We have tried to give clear, albeit brief, explanations of the details of each case. Instructors may choose to omit the more complex cases, which are deliberately written at a level that will stretch most students' understanding.

We chose to present mainly autopsy cases, as this type of case enabled us to consider the course of disease throughout a patient's life. In addition, more information is available at autopsy than from biopsy specimens, permitting a more detailed consideration of the effects of disease throughout the body. The use of autopsy cases also introduces some biases. We have tended to neglect surgical specimens, which form a much larger fraction of a typical pathologist's workload than do autopsies. Most patients do not have the very complicated disease courses that are illustrated in these cases. Also, modern medicine *is* effective for many patients. Even if they eventually die with or of their chronic diseases, most patients experience many therapeutic successes.

We have not included any pediatric cases in this book. We felt that the 10 or so pediatric cases that we might have included would not do justice to this large discipline. We hope to write a similar pediatric casebook at some later date.

Nancy Standler, M.D., Ph.D.
Bernard Klionsky, M.D.

ACKNOWLEDGMENTS

A work of this kind cannot be done without the help of many individuals, all of whose contributions we appreciate. We particularly thank the pathologists and their staff associates with the hospitals of the University of Pittsburgh. We also thank the editorial staff at Churchill Livingstone.

CONTENTS

III. HEMATOLOGY /53

Other cases pertaining to hematology: Case 1 (coagulopathy), Case 4 (drug-induced hematological problems), Case 6 (disseminated intravascular coagulation), Case 8 (hypercoagulability), Case 13 (occult lymphoma), Case 16 (mediastinal lymphadenopathy), Case 19 (idiopathic thrombocytopenic purpura), Case 22 (polycythemia), Case 24 (coagulopathy), Case 26 (lymphoma), Case 27 (lymphoma), Case 35 (myelophthisic anemia), Case 36 (disseminated intravascular coagulation)

IV. RESPIRATORY SYSTEM /79

Other cases pertaining to the respiratory system: Case 1 (multiple respiratory complications), Case 3 (restrictive lung disease), Case 4 (interstitial pulmonary fibrosis), Case 6 (emphysema, pulmonary hypertension), Case 8 (pulmonary emboli), Case 9 (amyloidosis), Case 10 (AIDS), Case 11 (aspergillosis, sarcoidosis), Case 12 (aspergillosis), Case 17 (tracheostomy), Case 18 (aspiration), Case 19 (ARDS), Case 20 (pulmonary emboli, pulmonary metastases), Case 24 (pulmonary edema), Case 26 (pneumonia), Case 29 (amyotrophic lateral sclerosis), Case 31 (multiple respiratory complications), Case 33 (staphylococcal pneumonia with abscess), Case 35 (multiple respiratory complications), Case 36 (adult respiratory distress syndrome)

V. GASTROINTESTINAL TRACT /105

Other cases pertaining to the gastrointestinal tract: Case 1 (ulcerative colitis), Case 2 (appendiceal abscess), Case 3 (esophageal stricture), Case 4 (ischemic necrosis of bowel), Case 9 (amyloidosis), Case 11 (thrush), Case 15 (diverticular disease), Case 16 (peptic ulcer disease), Case 21 (abdominal trauma), Case 22 (multiple bowel complications), Case 23 (ischemic colitis, diverticulitis), Case 24 (gastrointestinal hemorrhage), Case 29 (amyotrophic lateral sclerosis)

VI. LIVER AND PANCREAS /129

Other cases of interest pertaining to the liver and pancreas: Case 1 (liver failure, pancreatitis), Case 10 (hepatitis), Case 15 (α1-antitrypsin deficiency), Case 16 (hepatitis, hepatic metastases), Case 25 (polycystic liver disease)

VII. URINARY SYSTEM /153

SYSTEMIC DISEASE

1 MULTIORGAN FAILURE IN A PATIENT WITH HISTORY OF ULCERATIVE COLITIS

Key Words | *ulcerative colitis, colectomy, multiorgan failure*

CASE

The patient was a 37-year-old man with a 15-year history of ulcerative colitis who had required total colectomy four years previously (Fig. 1-1). Immediately postoperatively, the superior mesenteric artery thrombosed. The resultant infarction of the small bowel required resection and jejunostomy.[1] After this, the patient had recurrent pancreatitis and pancreatic insufficiency, which required enzyme replacement therapy. The patient had a three-year history of elevated liver function tests and a ten-month history of jaundice and pruritus. The results of four liver biopsies were negative except for fat infiltration. Possible causes of the liver disease included cholestasis secondary to hyperalimentation, sclerosing cholangitis, and extrahepatic obstruction.[2] The patient required significant pain medication because of his multiple surgeries and recurrent pancreatitis. Drug-seeking behavior had been noted in the past and on current admission.[3]

The patient was admitted to the hospital and evaluated for possible multiple organ transplantation. At the time of admission, he was in reasonably good health except for mild anemia and some jaundice. He remained in the program waiting for a suitable transplant for several months.[4] He spent approximately one week at home on a pass. He

DISCUSSION

1. Ulcerative colitis is an inflammatory disease of the bowel that may progress rapidly or slowly to involve larger regions of the intestine. It is not unusual for patients with ulcerative colitis to have a total colectomy either to control the symptoms or to reduce the risk of cancer. This patient had the unfortunate postoperative complication of infarction of most of his remaining bowel. Following the resection of the necrotic bowel, the patient had only a fraction of the normal absorptive surface and could no longer digest and absorb a normal diet. Patients with short bowels are particularly vulnerable to malnutrition.

2. Although the precise cause of this patient's pancreatitis is not clear, the pancreas does not function normally in patients with short bowels. This patient's history of chronic pancreatitis requiring enzyme replacement therapy may thus have been related to his short bowel syndrome. He also had a number of possible reasons for developing liver dysfunction. Ulcerative colitis is associated with fatty infiltration, chronic active hepatitis, pericholangitis, sclerosing cholangitis, and bile duct carcinoma. Cholestasis can occur because the normal circulation of cholesterol and bile salts is badly impaired in patients with short bowels. Sclerosing cholangitis is a disease of unknown cause characterized by sclerosis of intrahepatic bile ducts.

3

CASE

then developed a two-day history of increasing epigastric pain, fever, chills, weakness, and fluctuating mental status. Since the serum amylase level was increased, the clinical impression was acute pancreatitis, with a second possibility of sepsis.[5] Two days later, the patient complained of shortness of breath, increasing abdominal pain, and sputum production. The clinical impression was deterioration of pulmonary status; possible causes included pneumonia, fluid overload, and adult respiratory distress syndrome from pancreatitis or other causes. He was treated with antibiotics for possible hospital-acquired and community-acquired pneumonia. Sputum cultures grew normal flora, and a direct fluorescent-antibody test for *Legionella* was negative.[6]

Several days later, the patient became hypotensive. He appeared to have high-output heart failure, presumably related to the combination of sepsis or pancreatitis, anemia, and pulmonary dysfunction.[7] Despite pressor therapy, he became oliguric and had rising blood urea nitrogen and creatinine levels. The renal failure was considered to be possibly secondary to hypotension. Another possibility was acute tubular necrosis secondary to angiogram dye. The patient had been exposed to the dye during a pulmonary angiogram that was performed to rule out the possibility of pulmonary embolism. He required transfusions to keep his hematocrit above 30% (normal, 40 to 52%). His pulmonary, renal, abdominal, and cardiovascular problems all continued to worsen. The clinical impression was that the patient was in multisystem failure as a result of sepsis, although no source was identified.[8]

The patient was found dead two weeks after he developed fever and respiratory distress. Autopsy results confirmed multiorgan failure. Both the ileum and colon had been surgically removed. The liver showed fibrosis, centrilobular necrosis, and cholestasis. Chronic severe pancreatitis with fat necrosis, pancreatic insufficiency, and multiple pseudocyst formation was present (Fig. 1-2).[9] The heart showed fibrinous pericarditis with extensive hemorrhage. The meninges showed subarachnoid and subdural hemorrhage. Acute bronchopneumonia and organizing interstitial pneumonia with abscess formation and probable sepsis were

DISCUSSION

3. Drug-seeking behavior in a patient with a long history of chronic pain with acute exacerbations is not unusual. Both psychological and physiological dependence may have contributed.
4. Many chronic diseases can produce a mild anemia. With the exception of anemia and liver dysfunction, this patient was in quite good health considering the degree to which his gastrointestinal function had been compromised. For this reason, he was considered to be a suitable candidate for multiorgan transplantation. The transplantation would presumably have involved liver, pancreas, small intestine, and colon.
5. Acute pancreatitis and sepsis can appear similar clinically. Amylase is a pancreatic enzyme whose serum levels rise when the pancreas is damaged.
6. When there are many possible causes of respiratory difficulties, it may be difficult to determine the specific cause. Unfortunately, rational therapy usually requires an accurate diagnosis. *Legionella* causes a serious pneumonia. Fluorescent-antibody staining of sputum provides a method of detecting this organism, which is difficult to culture.
7. In high-output heart failure, tissue oxygenation is inadequate despite the large volumes of blood being pumped by the heart. Factors that can contribute to poor perfusion include low blood pressure, anemia, and a dysfunctional pulmonary system. These factors may have acted synergistically in this patient.
8. This patient's pattern of multiorgan failure became clearly established when renal failure also developed. Although the patient was initially able to maintain reasonable health in the absence of extraneous stress, he was very vulnerable to additional stress. This patient's terminal course was initiated by what was apparently an episode of acute pancreatitis followed by pneumonia. Many other processes, such as other infections, trauma, myocardial infarction, or overhydration, might have initiated a similar terminal course. In general, once substantial disease occurs in multiple organ systems, it becomes increasingly difficult to reverse a progressively worsening course. The partial or complete failure of each organ tends to put additional stress on the remaining systems. The low hematocrit may have been due to a combination of occult bleeding and inadequate marrow production. Sources of sepsis may be difficult to identify in patients with multiorgan failure because of the number

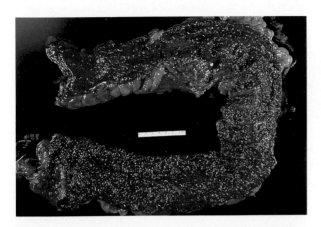

Fig. 1-1. Ulcerative colitis (gross specimen, from another case). The entire length of colonic mucosa has been denuded by ulcerative colitis to produce a bright-red, inflamed surface that bleeds easily. Such mucosa cannot perform its normal absorptive role in digestion. The walls of the colon are relatively unaffected.

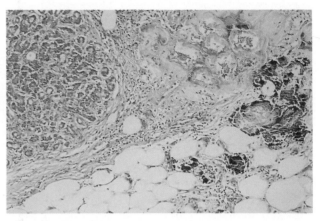

Fig. 1-2. Acute and chronic pancreatitis (low power photomicrograph, hematoxylin and eosin). Healthy pancreatic acini and adipose tissue are shown on the left. A mixed inflammatory exudate, indicating acute and chronic pancreatitis, is visible in the fibrous tissue in the center of the field. The destruction of pancreatic acini (*above right*) can occur in both acute and chronic pancreatitis. Characteristic of chronic pancreatitis is the deposition of calcium soaps in injured adipose tissue to form large, dark deposits (*far right*).

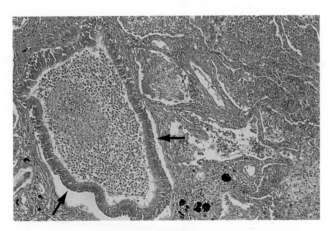

Fig. 1-3. Bronchopneumonia (low power photomicrograph, hematoxylin and eosin, from another case). A bronchus (*arrows*) and adjacent alveoli are filled with an acute inflammatory exudate.

CASE

present (Fig. 1-3). Chronic pyelonephritis and chronic bronchitis were also found. There was no residual evidence of ulcerative colitis. A striking finding was the presence of abundant macrophages in the spleen, liver, bone, lymph nodes, and lung. Some were foamy, and some contained iron pigment. Blood, spleen, and lung cultures were sterile. In summary, the cause of death was considered to be sepsis and bronchopneumonia, with damage to many organs contributing to the patient's debilitated state.[10]

DISCUSSION

of abnormal findings that are present. Patients should be examined for possible sources such as abscess or other infections in the gastrointestinal tract, pneumonia or abscess in the lungs, urinary tract infection, and skin sources such as a decubitus ulcer.

9. Sclerosing cholangitis is excluded by the hepatic findings observed at autopsy. Cholestasis secondary to hyperalimentation and extrahepatic obstruction secondary to pancreatitis are both consistent with the autopsy findings. Pseudocysts can form in chronic pancreatitis secondary to obstruction of pancreatic ducts. Fat necrosis occurs when the pancreatitis causes release of active pancreatic enzymes into the peripancreatic fat. Chronic pancreatitis is distinguished from acute pancreatitis by increased fibrosis and cellular infiltrate consistent with chronic inflammation.

10. Fibrinous pericarditis can occur secondary to uremia; it did not reflect infection of the pericardium in this patient. Hemorrhage in the pericardium and meninges was the result of disseminated intravascular coagulation associated with the patient's sepsis. The subarachnoid and subdural hemorrhage was secondary to the patient's bleeding diathesis. The lung abscess provides a possible source of sepsis with secondary hypotension and disseminated intravascular coagulation. The bronchopneumonia and organizing interstitial pneumonia explain the patient's respiratory difficulties. Chronic pyelonephritis was an unsuspected finding that might have been treated with antibiotics if identified earlier. Both the chronic pyelonephritis and the chronic bronchitis are additional sources of possible sepsis. The foamy macrophages are not readily explainable, but may have been secondary to the administration of fat emulsion mixtures during long-term hyperalimentation. Sterile culture indicates that the antibiotic therapy was appropriate. Once multiorgan failure begins, adequate control of infection is not always sufficient to allow a patient to survive.

Inflammatory Bowel Disease

Crohn's disease and ulcerative colitis are inflammatory diseases of the mucosa of the gastrointestinal tract. In pure form, the diseases are quite distinct. Crohn's disease produces patchy, penetrating lesions that usually involve principally the ileum. The lesions are granulomatous, and fistulas and strictures commonly form in the intestinal wall. In contrast, the lesions in ulcerative colitis are superficial, do not form granulomas, involve the colon and rectum preferentially, and produce inflammatory polyposis. In spite of what would appear to be clearly distinguishable features, many cases with intermediate properties occur. This problem occurs in part because an intestinal biopsy is typically small and samples only the mucosa and not the wall of the intestine. Consequently, it may not be possible to demonstrate the presence of granulomas and involvement of the muscle of the intestinal wall in the sampled tissue. The diagnostic problem is exacerbated if diagnosis is delayed until both the small intestine and colon are involved in the disease process. Additionally, the diseases share a number of common features. Although the onset of symptoms may occur at any age, childhood and young adulthood are typical ages of onset for both diseases. Both ulcerative colitis and Crohn's disease can impair absorption of nutrients. In severe cases, this can cause failure of growth and development of secondary sexual characteristics in children and adolescents. Both diseases sometimes occur in a single family. Both are associated in some patients with a variety of syndromes affecting other organ systems, including arthritis, dermatological manifestations, ocular inflammation, liver disease, pyelonephritis, renal stones, and amyloidosis.

Questions

1. Describe the clinical and pathological features of ulcerative colitis and Crohn's disease. How are these diseases similar? Different? What types of systemic manifestations can they have?
2. Describe this patient's medical history. What problems related to his ulcerative colitis, or its therapy, had he experienced? What organ systems were affected?
3. Why was he admitted to the hospital? What happened after he went home on a pass? Describe his subsequent hospital course. Why was he vulnerable to multiorgan failure? What was found at autopsy?

Selected Reading

Lake AM: Recognition and management of inflammatory bowel disease in children and adolescents. Curr Probl Pediatr 18:377–437, 1988.

Offenbartl K, Bengmark S: Intra-abdominal infections and gut origin sepsis. World J Surg 14:191–195, 1990.

Riis P: Inflammation as a diagnostic keystone and its clinical implications, exemplified by the inflammatory bowel diseases. Agents Actions 29:4–7, 1990.

Waxman K: Postoperative multiple organ failure. Crit Care Clin 3:429–440, 1987.

2 CEREBRAL HEMORRHAGE IN A PATIENT WITH SYSTEMIC LUPUS ERYTHEMATOSUS

Key Words | systemic lupus erythematosus, appendicitis, cerebral hemorrhage

CASE

The patient was a 29-year-old woman who had been diagnosed with systemic lupus erythematosus at age 12.[1] Since that time she had been treated with azathioprine and prednisone. She had also been treated with hydrochlorothiazide since diagnosis of diffuse proliferative glomerulitis at age 25. A left lateral ankle abscess secondary to vasculitis had required surgical drainage one year before her final admission.[2]

The patient was admitted to the hospital with a complaint of one and a half days of predominantly epigastric abdominal pain. Also, she complained of diarrhea and headache for the preceding few days. She was noted to have a fever (temperature, 39.1°C [normal, 37°C] rectally). The abdomen was soft and was not distended. Tenderness was present in the right lower quadrant.[3] The blood pressure was 134/70 mmHg (normal, 100 to 140/60 to 90 mmHg) with pulse 96/min (normal, 60 to 100/min) and respiratory rate of 20/min (normal 6 to 20/min). Serum creatinine was 1.5 mg/100 ml (normal, 0.5 to 1.4 mg/100 ml). The urine showed

DISCUSSION

1. This patient had had systemic lupus erythematosus for at least 17 years, and consequently might have many organ systems damaged by vasculitis. The diagnosis at age 12 was made at an earlier age than usual. Lupus is suspected when a girl or a young woman has symptoms of systemic disease that are not easily attributed to some other process. If this patient had been ill for several months at age 12 and had a rash and arthralgias, she would probably have been tested for antinuclear antibodies.

2. The immunosuppressive agent azathioprine is used in transplantation procedures, systemic lupus erythematosus, rheumatoid arthritis, and a number of other systemic inflammatory states. The corticosteroid prednisone reduces inflammation. Lupus slowly damages the kidneys, and renal failure is one of the most dreaded complications. The diuretic hydrochlorothiazide improves kidney function in the presence of renal disease. Tissue distal to a vascular lesion may have impaired perfusion and is consequently vulnerable to infection.

3. The patient's symptoms suggest that she had an in-

9

CASE

proteinuria (2+) and nonhemolyzed blood. Air/fluid levels on the right side were observed by abdominal radiography. There appeared to be free air throughout the abdominal films. The clinical impression was of an acute abdomen of unknown cause, possibly appendiceal abscess.[4]

The patient's appendix, which showed necrotizing vasculitis, was removed during exploratory laparotomy. On the second postoperative day, the patient noticed weakness of her left hand and numbness of her right hand. A myelogram was negative. Blood pressure was 150/100 mmHg. The clinical impression was that these neurological problems were central in nature and were possibly due to a cerebral infarction.[5] The blood pressure rose to 205/110 mmHg four days after admission, despite the use of strong diuretics. Serum complement factor C3 was 51.5 mg/100 ml (normal, 83 to 177 mg/100 ml) and had decreased from 76 mg/100 ml three months earlier.[6]

Two days later, the patient became uncooperative. She showed a decrease in her leg strength. There was obvious bilateral upper extremity weakness with flexor contracture. Four days after rising, her blood pressure returned to 134/88 mmHg. Her temperature was 37.4°C. The clinical impression was that she had a left parietal hematoma.[7] The next day she responded to deep pain by adopting a decerebrate posture. A left parietal occipital craniotomy was performed, and a hemorrhagic infarct with blood clot was removed from the left occipital and parietal lobes. Postoperatively, there was no spontaneous movement. She continued to respond to pain by adopting a decerebrate posture. One week after the craniotomy, she had evidence of brainstem dysfunction. Her neurological conditions continued without improvement. The patient became asystolic and was pronounced dead approximately two and one half weeks after the appendectomy.[8]

At autopsy, the patient was found to have generalized acute necrotizing arteritis and old healed arteritis in most of the organs (Fig. 2-1). The kidneys showed chronic diffuse proliferative glomerulonephritis with extensive glomerular scarring (Fig. 2-2). Postmortem immunofluores-

DISCUSSION

fection. Pain in the appendix is often referred to the periumbilical area. Local signs in the lower right quadrant are produced when the peritoneum becomes inflamed. Tenderness in the lower right quadrant supported the possibility of appendiceal or cecal involvement. The absence of guarding with a soft, nondistended abdomen suggests that generalized peritonitis had not yet developed.

4. Clinical evidence of glomerular disease is provided by the patient's high-normal serum creatinine, urine protein, and nonhemolyzed blood in urine. The presence of free air and air/fluid levels in the abdominal radiographs suggests that perforation may have occurred. Exploratory laparotomy was a reasonable next step to define and, if possible, correct the gastrointestinal problem.

5. Necrotizing vasculitis in the appendix was consistent with the history of systemic lupus erythematosus and consequent risk of vasculitis. The patient's neurological symptoms figured prominently in her course and produced a clinical picture that was difficult to interpret. Lupus-induced vasculitis in the brain with the risk of subsequent hemorrhage and infarction was one clinical possibility, although later autopsy findings ruled this out. The combination of motor and sensory symptoms in opposite hands suggests that the patient might have spinal cord disease, since this is the level at which a single relatively small lesion might produce both symptoms. However, the patient's myelogram was normal. This would rule out a cord lesion, leaving the possibility that an infarction or hemorrhage had occurred as a complication of surgery.

6. The abrupt rise in blood pressure occurred for unknown reasons, possibly either acute exacerbation of the glomerulonephritis or central nervous system damage by hemorrhage, infarct, or edema. During active phases of systemic lupus erythematosus, serum complement factors are often decreased secondary to consumption in areas of vasculitis.

7. Changes in mental status and weakness in the extremities suggest progressing neurological dysfunction. Lupus-induced vasculitis in the meninges can produce hemorrhage. The risk of hemorrhage is markedly increased in a patient with severe hypertension.

8. The decerebrate posture in response to pain indicates

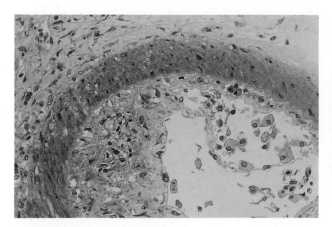

Fig. 2-1. Endothelial proliferation (kidney, high power photomicrograph, toluidine blue). Endothelial proliferation has narrowed the lumen of this small artery. Similar damage was observed in many of this patient's intrarenal vessels and was probably a consequence of the hypertension that can accompany systemic lupus erythematosus.

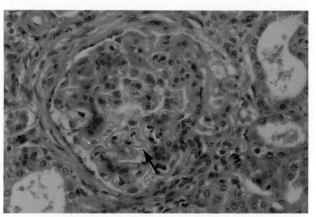

Fig. 2-2. Diffuse proliferative glomerulonephritis (kidney, high power photomicrograph, hematoxylin and eosin). The glomerulus in the center of this field shows such a marked cellular proliferation that the space in Bowman's capsule is visible only as a thin white ring separating the glomerular tufts from the fibrous outside wall of the glomerulus. Adhesions can be seen between the glomerular epithelial cells and Bowman's capsule along the right edge of the glomerulus. Most of the glomerular capillary beds have markedly thickened walls. In only a few places *(arrow)* does the tuft appear more normal.

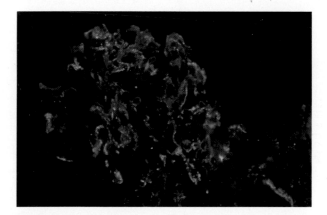

Fig. 2-3. IgM deposits in a glomerulus (kidney, high power photomicrograph, immunofluorescence technique for IgM). IgM deposits in the mesangium and capillary wall show as fluorescent green granular deposits. Further immunological studies demonstrated that this patient's glomeruli also contained a variety of other immunoglobulins and complement factors.

CASE

cence studies of kidney tissue showed a typical pattern for diffuse proliferative glomerulonephritis of systemic lupus erythematosus with IgG, IgM, IgA, C1q, and C3 staining in a granular distribution in the glomerular mesangium (Fig. 2-3). Electron microscopy of kidney tissue showed discrete electron-dense deposits in mesangial, intramembranous, and subendothelial locations. Focal mesangial cell interposition with double-contour glomerular basement membrane was seen in capillary loops.[9]

Contrary to expectation, evidence of lupus vasculitis was not found in the central nervous system. Grossly, the brain showed multiple hemorrhages in the left frontoparietal cortex, basal ganglia, and right middle frontal gyrus; epidural hematoma; subarachnoid hemorrhage; and diffuse encephalomalacia. Histological studies demonstrated multiple focal, recent infarcts in the cortex, basal ganglia, cerebellum, and pons. A ruptured small aneurysm was found in the anterior vertebral artery, and it was thought that perhaps the patient's left parieto-occipital intracerebral hematoma was a consequence of rupture of a similar aneurysm.[10]

DISCUSSION

severe, and probably irreversible, dysfunction of higher brain centers. Removal of the clot potentially improved neurological dysfunction related to edema or pressure effects. Unfortunately, if tissue necrosis has occurred, the neurological defects may not be reversible.

9. Since lupus-induced arteritis is a focal process that subsequently heals, lesions of different apparent ages are found throughout the body. Lupus erythematosus can produce the variety of renal findings illustrated in this case. The prominent immunofluorescent staining for antibodies and complement factors reflects their role in the pathophysiology of lupus renal disease.

10. The patient's severe hypertension produced widespread and devastating central nervous system hemorrhage. The basal ganglia, pons, and cerebellum are particularly vulnerable to hypertensive hemorrhage and were damaged in this patient. Hemorrhage from preexisting vascular malformations or aneurysms is also exacerbated in severe hypertension. This may have been the cause of the left parietal hematoma. Once hemorrhage begins, a pattern of progressive damage to the nervous system can result as edema and compression of central nervous system structures cause increasing damage. The patient's fall in blood pressure, if the rise was originally central in character, may have occurred as the brainstem was beginning to die.

Systemic Lupus Erythematosus

Systemic lupus erythematosus is a disease of young to middle-aged women, with 90% of the cases occurring in women between the ages of 12 and 40. More than 80% of patients survive ten years or more. When death does occur, common causes are infection, renal failure, gastrointestinal hemorrhage or infarction, and central nervous system disease.

Only a few manifestations of lupus are typically present in a given patient. Depending upon exactly which sites are involved, the clinical presentation of lupus is widely variable. Most of the symptoms associated with systemic lupus erythematosus can be considered to be manifestations of three processes: small vessel vasculitis, serositis, and deposition of immune complexes in tissue parenchyma. The endothelium of small arteries and arterioles becomes damaged, possibly by deposition in the vessel wall of complexes formed of DNA and anti-DNA immunoglobin together with complement, and subsequently reacts by a concentric proliferation that narrows the vessel lumen. The necrotizing vasculitis so produced can be widespread and may cause ischemia in many organs. Kidney, skin, and central nervous system are most commonly involved. Also characteristic of lupus is a polyserositis associated with fibrin deposition that can cause joint, peritoneal, and pleuropericardial symptoms. Arthritis is the most common symptom associated with lupus. Similar changes involving the pericardium or pleural cavity first produce inflammation and fibrin deposition and, when present chronically, may eventually lead to partial or complete obliteration of the serosal cavity by scar tissue.

The manifestations include a number of rashes (a butterfly-shaped rash on the nose and cheek, a discoid rash, photosensitivity, and oral ulcers); arthritis and serositis; renal disease with persistent proteinuria or cellular casts; and neurological disease including seizures and psychosis. Hematological disease can be present, including hemolytic anemia, leukopenia, lymphopenia, and thrombocytopenia. A variety of immunological manifestations may include LE cells, false-positive VDRL on test for syphilis, and antibodies to DNA antibody and smooth muscle cells.

Questions

1. What is systemic lupus erythematosus? What are its clinical manifestations? Which manifestations did this patient experience before her final admission? How was she treated?

2. What were the patient's presenting complaints at her final admission? What was found on physical examination? What did laboratory studies show? What differential diagnosis was considered? What was found at exploratory laparotomy? How was the patient's appendiceal disease related to her lupus?

3. What problems did the patient experience postoperatively? Describe her changing neurological status. What was thought to be the cause of her neurological problems? How were these problems treated? Was the treatment successful? Describe the autopsy findings.

Selected Reading

Denburg JA, Denburg SD, Carbotte RM et al: Nervous system involvement in systemic lupus erythematosus. Isr J Med Sci 24:754–758, 1988.

Hughes GR: Systemic lupus erythematosus. Postgrad Med J 64:517–521, 1988.

Tan EM: Antinuclear antibodies: diagnostic markers for autoimmune diseases and probes for cell biology. Adv Immunol 44:93–151, 1989.

3 SYSTEMIC SCLEROSIS

Key Words | *systemic sclerosis, esophageal stricture, skin ulcers*

CASE

The patient was a 32-year-old woman whose medical problems were attributable to progressive systemic sclerosis, diagnosed seven years earlier. At that time she first noted swelling of the right hand, which progressed over a few days to involve both hands. She then noted pain and blue discoloration of all fingers. Two months later she developed full Raynaud's phenomenon with triphasic color change and excruciating pain.[1] The erythrocyte sedimentation rate at that time was 70 mm/h (normal, <20 mm/h), antinuclear antibody was positive at a 1:2,500 dilution, and rheumatoid factor was positive at a 1:5,000 dilution. The entire maternal side of the patient's family had had rheumatoid arthritis and osteoarthritis.[2]

In the seven years between diagnosis of systemic sclerosis and final admission, the patient developed an extensive list of problems attributable to systemic sclerosis. She had multiple telangiectasias on her face, chest, and hands. The skin became markedly thickened, and extensive dermal fibrosis on the palms forced the fingers into flexure contraction (sclerodactyly). Impairment of circulation to the fingers, manifested by Raynaud's phenomenon, caused multiple digital ulcers. The patient had also been troubled by abscesses on the buttocks.[3] She had an esophageal stricture that had required dilation every one to three months for the preceding few years. She had a tendency to vomit during the period before dilation of the stricture. She had pain in both wrists, knees, ankles, elbows, and shoulders. A wrist fusion was performed six months before final admission because of rupture of the extensor tendons, wrist drop, and osteomyelitis. She had

DISCUSSION

1. Progressive systemic sclerosis is characterized by damage to small arterioles and deposition of excessive amounts of collagen throughout the body. In some patients, vasospasm of the small arteries in the hand occurs in response to cold or emotional stimuli. The spasm can produce severe pain and characteristic color changes as the skin of the fingers changes from white to blue to red. This cluster of symptoms is called *Raynaud's disease* when it occurs idiopathically. The term *Raynaud's phenomenon* is used when the symptoms are secondary to one of a wide variety of underlying disorders that damage vessel walls. Systemic sclerosis commonly presents with either swollen hands or Raynaud's phenomenon.

2. An increased erythrocyte sedimentation rate is a nonspecific indicator of inflammation. It is often related to increased fibrinogen or γ-globulin in the serum. The positive antinuclear antibody and rheumatoid factor suggest that a disease with an autoimmune component was present. As discussed in the pathophysiology section, systemic sclerosis appears to be related to other autoimmune diseases. The patient's positive family history for rheumatoid arthritis suggests a familial predisposition for autoimmune diseases with an arthritic component, such as systemic lupus erythematosus or this patient's systemic sclerosis.

3. This case illustrates the wide range of tissue damage that can occur in systemic sclerosis. Telangiectasias are spots visible on the skin above clusters of dilated small blood vessels. They occur on the face and hands in many patients with systemic sclerosis. In modern usage, the term *scleroderma* usually refers specifically to the thickening of the skin that occurs in systemic sclerosis and related conditions. The sclerodactyly

CASE

fatigue and shortness of breath. Pulmonary function tests performed one year earlier were consistent with moderately severe restrictive lung disease.[4] Myositis, diagnosed based on increased creatine phosphokinase levels, had been present for five years and had been treated with prednisone. The patient had Sjögren's syndrome with chronic dry eyes treated with artificial tears, dry mouth with occasional soreness, and vaginal irritation. She had complained of having to strain to empty the bladder and of having a slight increase in urination at night. Creatinine clearance at the time of her final admission was 50 ml/min (normal, 80 to 120 ml/min). Electrocardiographic studies showed incomplete right bundle branch block with occasional premature atrial contractions. The patient also had a hypochromic, microcytic anemia.[5]

The patient was admitted to the hospital for treatment of four buttock ulcers. There was extensive calcinosis in the subcutaneous tissues near the ulcers. These wounds had been present for about six weeks and had been treated with cephalosporins and emollient cream. After admission the buttock wounds were treated with dressings and chloramphenicol.[6] The anemia was treated with blood transfusions and oral ferrous sulfate. The patient's hospital course was complicated by the development of what was apparently an aspiration pneumonia. The pneumonia was thought to have been caused by vomiting secondary to esophageal stricture. She was still on steroid therapy for myositis. Three weeks after admission, the patient developed bradycardia with complete heart block and died.[7]

At autopsy the cause of death was considered to be multiple infections, respiratory failure, and shock, probably due to sepsis. The multiple infections included decubitus ulcers, extensive lobar pneumonia and bronchopneumonia, and an unsuspected subacute bacterial endocarditis.[8] Extensive dermal fibrosis was present. Sclerodactyly involved the hands, forcing the fingers into flexion contraction and limiting their range of motion (Figs. 3-1 and 3-2). Organizing infarctions were

DISCUSSION

that is produced when scleroderma involves the palms and fingers is very characteristic of advanced systemic sclerosis. Tissue, often in the skin of the fingertips, that is distal to involved arterioles may suffer ischemic damage. Such damage in the skin leads to the formation of ulcers that heal only with difficulty.

4. Although any portion of the gastrointestinal tract may be affected, the esophagus is particularly vulnerable. Stricture can occlude the lower esophageal sphincter. Repeated mechanical dilation (a painful process) may be required to permit passage of food from the esophagus to the stomach. The involvement of this patient's joints by disease was unusually pronounced and may have been related to her familial tendency to rheumatoid arthritis. Inflammation will weaken tendons, and spontaneous ruptures can occur. Unfortunately, such rupture is almost impossible to repair in patients in whom the underlying disease process continues, because the involved tissue will not heal. Fatigue is a common nonspecific symptom in patients with inflammatory disease. The patient's pulmonary symptoms and findings reflected fibrosis in the lungs.

5. The inflammatory process can also involve muscle. Fibrosis in salivary and tear glands occurs in a few patients and causes Sjögren's syndrome. The kidney is very sensitive to damage to arterioles. The reason for the patient's bladder problems was not clear but might have reflected either myositis or fibrosis around the urethra (neither was specifically noted at autopsy). Extensive fibrosis in the heart can cause congestive heart failure. Focal fibrosis can cause arrhythmias if the conducting system of the heart is interrupted. The patient's anemia may have been due to either iron deficiency or chronic inflammatory disease.

6. The buttocks are particularly vulnerable to the formation of decubitus ulcers. The vulnerability is due to the combination of the local hypoxia that can occur with prolonged sitting or lying, which is exacerbated in this case by the vascular disease of systemic sclerosis, and the availability of a large variety of skin and gastrointestinal bacteria. The damaged subcutaneous tissue then forms a convenient surface and appropriate pH conditions for the precipitation of cal-

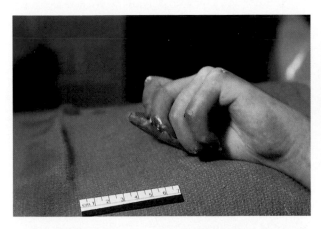

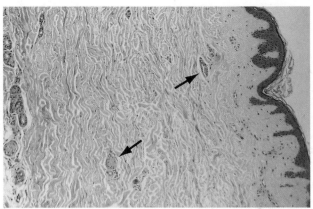

Fig. 3-1. Scleroderma involving hand (gross photograph). Skin involved with scleroderma typically becomes markedly thickened and less flexible. This patient's hand shows tightly-stretched skin with gangrenous fingers.

Fig. 3-2. Scleroderma affecting skin (low power photomicrograph, hematoxylin and eosin). The epidermis is on the far right. The subcutaneous tissue shows replacement of normal fat with a wide band of dense collage in which are entrapped a few normal structures *(arrows)* such as blood vessels and sweat glands.

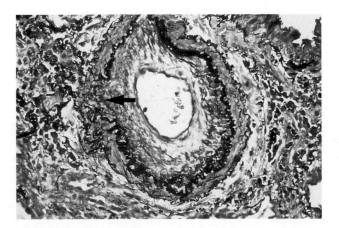

Fig. 3-3. Vessel damage in systemic sclerosis (lung, high power photomicrograph, elastic tissue stain, from another case). Disruption of elastic tissue *(arrow)* and endothelial proliferation are seen in this small artery. Such vascular changes occur locally in systemic sclerosis. (Courtesy of Dr. S. Yousem, Department of Pathology, University of Pittsburgh, Pittsburgh, Pennsylvania.)

CASE

present on all distal fingers and toes. The esophageal muscles showed fibrosis and atrophy. Microscopic examination of synovial membrane showed extensive fibrosis with loss of synovial lining cells and fibrin deposition on the surface. Skeletal muscles showed nonspecific myopathic changes.[9]

There was a striking pattern of end-organ ischemic necrosis: digital infarcts, cortical necrosis of the kidneys, and marked centrilobular hepatic necrosis. The renal and hepatic lesions were far more severe than the usual renal and hepatic necrosis of terminal shock. The lesions probably resulted from hypoperfusion and chronic arterial damage due to systemic sclerosis.[10]

DISCUSSION

cium. The resulting crystals further damage the skin. Decubitus ulcers may be difficult to treat because a variety of bacteria typically infect the wounds.

7. Patients who have difficulty in swallowing are vulnerable to aspiration pneumonia. Infections in a patient who is immunosuppressed because of steroid therapy tend to be much more dangerous than those in patients with normal immune systems. The bradycardia leading to complete heart block was probably the consequence of progressive damage by the systemic sclerosis to the cardiac conducting system.

8. Patients with multiple known infections often develop additional infections whose existence is not clinically suspected because preexisting disease appears to offer an adequate explanation of physical and laboratory findings.

9. All of these findings were known before the patient's death. Diseased skeletal muscle only rarely shows specific changes that can be associated with a single pathological process. Involvement of synovial membrane in systemic sclerosis is somewhat more specific, and biopsy of synovial membrane is sometimes helpful in making the diagnosis.

10. Many focal lesions in the circulatory system, particularly those involving smaller vessels, are difficult to confirm histologically because the appropriate sites in the vessels are often not sampled in the histological sections studied (Fig. 3-3).

Systemic Sclerosis

Systemic sclerosis is a complex disease whose pathophysiology is still not completely elucidated. In a variety of organs, the endothelial lining of some arterioles can become so thickened that a small distal infarction is produced. The arteriolar defects tend to be focal and, because of sampling problems, are not always found during microscopic examination. Collagen deposition characteristically occurs in the dermis to produce marked thickening coupled with atrophy of the overlying epidermis. Similar fibrosis can also occur in many other organs including the lungs, kidneys, gastrointestinal tract, heart, and the synovium of joints. This excessive collagen deposition appears to reflect abnormal fibroblast metabolism. Systemic sclerosis also has an autoimmune component with antibodies directed against nuclear constituents, particularly the nonhistone protein ScL-70 and centromeres. The relationship between the autoimmune process and the pronounced fibrosis may involve the production by collagen-sensitized lymphocytes of lymphokines that stimulate fibroblasts.

Systemic sclerosis is one of several conditions that

are sometimes referred to as scleroderma. Scleroderma that has no systemic involvement and is confined to localized regions of the skin occurs in two forms. Linear scleroderma occurs in children and is characterized by a linear patch of scleroderma on an extremity. Morphea is characterized by localized thickened patches of the skin. Another variant, the CREST variant, usually has a mild course with little systemic involvement. It is characterized by *c*alcinosis, *R*aynaud's phenomenon, *e*sophageal dysfunction, *s*clerodactyly, and *t*elangiectasias.

Questions

1. Discuss the pathophysiology of systemic sclerosis. What happens to some arterioles in systemic sclerosis? What are the consequences of abnormal fibroblast metabolism?

2. Which organs besides the skin can be involved in systemic sclerosis? Is scleroderma identical to systemic sclerosis? What is morphea? Linear scleroderma? The CREST variant?

3. Which organs were affected by scleroderma in this patient? What symptoms did she experience? Which laboratory findings were abnormal? How did her systemic sclerosis lead to death? What was found at autopsy?

Selected Reading

Geppert T: Clinical features, pathogenic mechanisms, and new developments in the treatment of systemic sclerosis. Am J Med Sci 299:103–209, 1990.

Merlo A, Cohen S: Swallowing disorders. Annu Rev Med 39:17–28, 1988.

4 MULTIPLE ADVERSE DRUG REACTIONS

Key Words | drug toxicities, arrhythmias, pulmonary fibrosis

CASE

A 49-year-old man presented with a two-day history of ataxia and confusion. The patient had a nine-year history of idiopathic thrombocytopenic purpura that had been treated with splenectomy and prednisone. Two months before the final admission, platelet counts decreased to about 10,000/mm³ (normal, 150,000 to 450,000/mm³). The platelet count transiently increased to about 50,000/mm³ after treatment with vinblastine. The vinblastine therapy was discontinued when the patient developed neutropenia and fever.[1]

The patient had experienced a myocardial infarction several months before admission. Ventricular tachycardia and congestive heart failure had developed secondarily. The arrhythmia was refractory to conventional antiarrhythmic agents and was treated with amiodarone.[2] The congestive heart failure was treated with the cardiac stimulant digoxin, the vasodilator isosorbide dinitrate, the angiotensin-converting enzyme inhibitor captopril, and the diuretic furosemide. The patient also had a history of several years of hypertension, mild diabetes mellitus controlled by diet, and Cushing's syndrome. These problems were thought to be secondary to prednisone therapy.[3]

The patient was admitted to the hospital with a two-day history of ataxia, confusion, nausea, and tingling in his hands. Physical examination was notable for a buffalo hump at the base of the neck and bilateral basilar rales. Neurological examination revealed decreased memory, poor motor strength in the proximal muscles of all extremi-

DISCUSSION

1. Ataxia is a failure of muscular coordination that manifests as difficulty in walking or poorly coordinated walking. The combination of confusion and ataxia indicates that some process has involved physically distant regions of the central nervous system. Idiopathic thrombocytopenic purpura is an autoimmune condition in which antibodies are directed against platelets. Removal of the spleen limits phagocytosis of antibody-coated platelets. Prednisone impairs the immune response. Decreasing platelet counts suggest that the patient had an acute exacerbation of idiopathic thrombocytopenic purpura. Bleeding does not usually occur until the counts are less than 60,000/mm³. Vinblastine is a potent chemotherapeutic agent that is used in the treatment of leukemias and can also be used in smaller doses to limit lymphocyte production. It is a toxic drug, and adverse effects, including bone marrow suppression and fever, are common.

2. The myocardial infarction was probably unrelated to the patient's idiopathic thrombocytopenic purpura. Both arrhythmias and congestive heart failure are among the complications of myocardial infarction. Amiodarone is a particularly potent, but also a particularly toxic, antiarrhythmic medication.

3. Many patients with congestive heart failure are on multiple medications since drugs acting by different mechanisms can have an additive effect. In addition to the immunosuppressive effects, corticosteroids such as prednisone can modify the metabolism of lipids and sugar.

4. The reason for this patient's prominent neurological

21

CASE

ties, and poor performance of tasks such as touching finger to nose and heel to shin.[4] Hematological studies showed moderate anemia, moderate neutropenia, and mild thrombocytopenia. The serum creatinine level was somewhat elevated. A chest radiograph showed interstitial pulmonary fibrosis that had not been present several months previously (Fig. 4-1).[5]

The impression at admission was that many of the patient's problems were related to drug toxicity. The ataxia and apparent cerebellar change were thought to be related to amiodarone or vinblastine toxicity. The vinblastine treatment had been previously discontinued, and the amiodarone treatment was discontinued at the time of admission. Anemia and neutropenia were thought to be due to vinblastine toxicity. Interstitial pulmonary fibrosis was thought to be due to amiodarone toxicity.[6] Since the patient's arrhythmia was apparently intractable, he was scheduled to have an automatic defibrillator surgically implanted. Computed tomography of the head revealed a lacunar infarct in the central white matter of the right hemisphere.[7]

Before the scheduled surgery, the patient developed an acute decrease in the platelet count to 5,000/mm^3. This decrease was treated with Sando immunoglobulin. Acute respiratory failure fol-

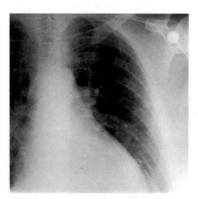

Fig. 4-1. Chest radiograph shows prominent interstitial abnormalities. The differential diagnosis included interstitial thickening secondary to drug therapy and early pulmonary edema.

DISCUSSION

symptoms was unclear. Acute onset of focal neurological symptoms tends to suggest processes such as infarction, hemorrhage, infection, or adverse reaction to some toxin or drug. Buffalo hump is a redistribution of fat to the base of the neck and is a common side effect of chronic steroid therapy. Bilateral basal rales occur in pulmonary edema secondary to congestive heart failure. Difficulty with pointing, coupled with ataxia, suggests cerebellar dysfunction. Poor motor strength in proximal muscles suggests motoneuron, peripheral nerve, or skeletal muscle disease. Memory loss was presumably related to loss of function in the cortex.

5. The anemia and neutropenia suggest that good control of the idiopathic thrombocytopenic purpura had caused excessive marrow suppression. Although severe anemia of acute onset can occasionally cause neurological dysfunction related to hypoxia, moderate anemia is not an adequate explanation for this patient's neurological findings. The somewhat elevated serum creatinine level raised the question of whether the patient was developing renal dysfunction. Interstitial pulmonary fibrosis of relatively acute onset is unusual; drug toxicity is a possible cause.

6. Amiodarone-induced neurotoxicity may manifest with a wide variety of symptoms including headache, nausea, myalgia, weakness, ataxia, paresthesias, depression, and hallucinations. Vinblastine-induced neurotoxicity occurs in about 5 to 20% of patients and may manifest as paresthesias, loss of deep-tendon reflexes, peripheral neuritis, depression, headache, and convulsions. The possibility that the two drugs were synergistically toxic should also be considered. If enough bone marrow has been damaged, removal of the offending drug may not reverse bone marrow suppression, or may reverse it only very slowly. Amiodarone has been associated with hypersensitivity pneumonitis and pulmonary fibrosis in a few patients, particularly those with preexisting pulmonary disease.

7. Under the circumstances of this patient's difficulties with medication coupled with intractable arrhythmias, the automatic defibrillator appeared to be a reasonable choice. The lacunar infarct could have accounted for proximal motor weakness but did not

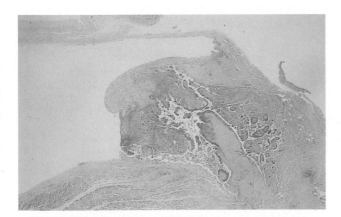

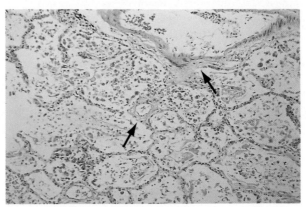

Fig. 4-2. Acute endocarditis (low power photomicrograph, hematoxylin and eosin). A large vegetation composed of inflammatory cells and eosinophilic, necrotic debris *(center of field)* lies at the junction of the thin valve leaflet *(above)* and the ventricular wall *(below)*. A valve leaflet can rupture if the necrosis extends through the leaflet. Emboli can be produced when a vegetation fragments as a result of hemodynamic stresses created by a beating heart.

Fig. 4-3. Chronic passive congestion (low power photomicrograph, hematoxylin and eosin). The alveoli are filled with macrophages, erythrocytes, and cellular debris. These changes are typically seen in chronic passive congestion. The interstitial pulmonary fibrosis diagnosed clinically is not prominent in this field, although there is some increase in the connective tissue around the blood vessels *(arrows)* and some thickening of alveolar walls.

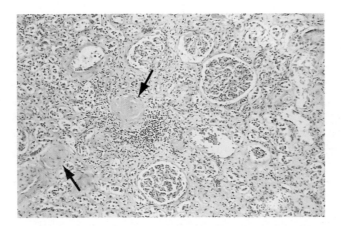

Fig. 4-4. Kidney (low power photomicrograph, hematoxylin and eosin). Several vessels, probably arterioles, are sclerosed *(arrows)*. One has a prominent lymphocytic infiltration at its margin. The glomeruli appear relatively normal or show some increase in cellularity. The interstitial areas show diffuse increase in fibrous tissue deposition around the tubules.

CASE

lowed; the differential diagnosis was pulmonary edema versus Arthus-type reaction to the immunoglobulin. The immunoglobulin treatment was discontinued, and the pulmonary edema resolved with diuresis and steroids.[8] The patient developed fever while in the intensive care unit. Blood cultures repeatedly grew *Staphylococcus aureus*. A sacral decubitus ulcer was thought to be the source of infection. An echocardiogram showed mitral and aortic regurgitation. Bacterial endocarditis was diagnosed and treated with oxacillin and gentamicin. Blood urea nitrogen and serum creatinine levels increased and urinary output decreased approximately two weeks after the initiation of antibiotic treatment. The patient was thought to have gentamicin toxicity, and therapy with this drug was discontinued, but renal failure continued to progress over the next week. Peritoneal dialysis was started.[9] The patient next developed pulmonary edema and changes in his mental status. Episodes of respiratory arrest and severe hypotension occurred despite therapy. The patient became markedly hypotensive, acidotic, and hypokalemic. He died shortly thereafter.[10]

Acute endocarditis was noted at autopsy (Fig. 4-2). Severe atherosclerosis was present, as were recent occlusive thromboemboli in the right and left anterior descending coronary arteries. An old myocardial infarction was observed. Interstitial consolidation involved the lungs diffusely (Fig. 4-3). Damage associated with hypotension and hypoxia included adult respiratory distress syndrome and ischemic necrosis in multiple gastrointestinal sites. The kidneys showed focal glomerulosis with diffuse interstitial cortical fibrosis and vascular sclerosis (Fig. 4-4). However, the reason for renal failure was not clearly documented at autopsy. Postmortem culture results were negative, indicating that antibiotics had controlled the endocarditis. Autopsy of the brain was not permitted by the family. The cause of death was considered to be acute myocardial infarction in a patient with idiopathic thrombocytopenic purpura, endocarditis, and renal failure.[11]

DISCUSSION

account for the cerebellar findings, so the possibility of drug-induced neurological damage remained.

8. Known bone marrow suppression coupled with an exacerbation of the idiopathic thrombocytopenic purpura could have produced the profound, and very dangerous, thrombocytopenia. Sando immunoglobulin is an intravenous immunoglobulin containing IgG antibodies collected from pooled human plasma. Sando immunoglobin is usually used in immunodeficiency disease. In idiopathic thrombocytopenic purpura, the immunoglobulin apparently reduces phagocytosis of platelets by blocking the Fc receptors on phagocytes. This patient's respiratory system was already vulnerable because of his history of pulmonary edema and interstitial fibrosis. Since Sando immunoglobin is a protein mixture, one hazard of therapy is the potential development of anaphylaxis.

9. Profound immunosuppression would be expected to leave this patient vulnerable to infection. Many bedridden patients develop decubitus ulcers. Endocarditis often involves valve leaflets and can consequently produce valvular insufficiency. Previously documented renal dysfunction may have increased this patient's vulnerability to drug-induced renal damage. The renal failure was most unfortunate, as from that point the patient followed a progressively worsening course.

10. Fluid retention due to diminished renal output led to pulmonary edema. A cyclical pattern of progressive damage to multiple organ systems had many causes: septicemia from the endocarditis; hypoxia due to pulmonary edema and fibrosis; metabolic, electrolyte, and pH disturbances related to renal failure; and damage to the previously damaged heart, leading to severe hypotension.

11. One of the striking features of this case is the large number of adverse drug effects suffered by this patient. The initial reason for his unusual vulnerability is not completely clear and may have reflected either simply bad luck or peculiarities of his metabolism. Many adverse drug reactions in healthier patients are subclinical. However, once multiple organs have been damaged by disease or other processes, the chance of a serious adverse reaction markedly increases.

Drug Toxicity

Few patients have as unfortunate a series of experiences with drugs as did this patient. We have included this case to illustrate that medications, particularly potent medications, are not always benign interventions that improve a patient's health. Dramatic cases such as this one can also lead a physician to conclude that the patient would have been better off without any intervention. Such a conclusion, however, neglects the fact that any of this patient's multiple life-threatening conditions, if left untreated, might have rapidly led to his death.

Some guidelines in the use of medications are helpful. The safety and well-being of the patient increase when problems are anticipated and avoided. Although some adverse reactions of drugs are idiosyncratic, many are not and are likely to be more common, severe, or dangerous in some patients than in others. Potential problems can often be anticipated by applying common sense and reading the entries about the drugs in package inserts, the *Physician's Desk Reference,* or a standard pharmacology text. It is usually wise to use as few drugs as possible and at as low a dose as possible. This implies that it may be advantageous to accept moderate rather than excellent control of a patient's symptoms in order to limit the toxicity of a potent drug. Most drugs should be avoided in pregnancy.

If possible, avoid multiple insults to an organ, since the patient's body is much less able to compensate for multiple insults than for a single insult. Other potential interactions that are not explicitly mentioned can often be deduced. If the metabolisms of two drugs share common steps (e.g., if both drugs are bound to serum protein or are degraded by the same microsomal system), either the effective concentration or the half-life of one or both drugs might be affected. Similarly, any conditions that a patient has that may alter drug metabolism or distribution should be considered in setting the dosage of the drugs. Renal or hepatic failure may limit drug excretion. Drug absorption may be impaired by gastrointestinal disease. Low serum albumin may reduce the amount of drug that is protein bound. Emaciation can reduce the amount of fat in which a lipid-soluble drug dissolves. Pulmonary edema may slow absorption of an aerosol drug. Hereditary or acquired conditions can limit the activity of an enzyme in the metabolism of a drug.

Questions

1. What is idiopathic thrombocytopenic purpura? Why is it dangerous? How was this patient's idiopathic thrombocytopenic purpura initially treated? Why was he treated with vinblastine? What cardiac conditions did this patient have? With what drugs were this patient's cardiac conditions treated?
2. Discuss the relationship of this patient's medications to the medical problems he experienced. What side effects of prednisone therapy were observed? What neurological and pulmonary problems did he experience? To which drugs might these problems have been related? What other drug-related problems did he experience?
3. Which organ systems were vulnerable in this patient? Why was each system vulnerable? What infections did this patient develop? How did they contribute to his death? What was found at autopsy?

Selected Reading

Coleman JW: Allergic reactions to drugs: current concepts and problems. Clin Exp Allergy 20:79–85, 1990.
Dukes MNG: Meyler's Side Effects of Drugs. 11th Ed. Elsevier, Amsterdam, 1988.

CARDIOVASCULAR SYSTEM

5 RUPTURED AORTIC ANEURYSM

Key Words | aortic aneurysm, atherosclerosis, cystic medial necrosis

CASE

A 62-year-old woman presented with abdominal pain. Eight years previously, the patient had undergone surgical repair of a dissecting thoracic aortic aneurysm. Four years later, she was noted to have increased serum creatinine levels. Angiography at that time demonstrated dissection of the remainder of the aorta (Fig. 5-1).[1] A right smaller lumen supplied an inferiorly displaced functioning right kidney and the celiac artery. The left large lumen supplied the iliac arteries. An intravenous pyelogram revealed decreased functioning of the left kidney. No intervention was performed because the patient was asymptomatic, the repair was surgically difficult, and there was concern about her renal function.[2]

The patient developed severe abdominal pain four years later that was considered to be due to rupture of the aneurysm. She was admitted to a community hospital, where a blood pressure of 70/52 mmHg (normal 100 to 140/60 to 90) and a heart rate of 80/min (normal, 60 to 100/min) were found. The patient was immediately transferred to a university hospital since her blood pressure continued to drop.[3] Physical examination in the emergency room revealed that she was pale and in acute distress. Her heart rate and rhythm were within normal limits. Pulses were 1+ in the upper extremities and present in the lower extremities as observed by the Doppler technique. The right lower extremity pulse was greater than the left.[4]

The abdomen was distended and without bowel sounds. A pulsatile mass was palpable. The

DISCUSSION

1. In general, thoracic aortic aneurysms tend to dissect without rupturing, whereas abdominal aortic aneurysms often rupture as they dissect. When no branches arise from the involved region, the damaged portion of the vessel is easily replaced with a synthetic graft. The surgical repair may not have been extended sufficiently. Alternatively, the same process that involved the earlier aneurysm may have produced an extension. The patient's increasing serum creatinine levels may have been due to renal damage caused by impaired renal blood flow.

2. Dissecting aneurysms sometimes involve a portion of the aorta containing major branches. When this happens, some branches may be supplied from the true aortic lumen and some branches from a false lumen. Surgical replacement of the damaged portion of the vessel then becomes technically difficult and may be associated with a high operative mortality rate. The decreased functioning of one kidney was presumably due to impaired perfusion secondary to atherosclerosis or the aortic dissection. The decision was to delay surgery since the risks of operating at that time were greater than the risks of spontaneous rupture.

3. The pain associated with a dissecting or rupturing aneurysm is characteristically described as severe, persistent, and ripping or tearing. The pain may be accompanied by dyspnea and must be distinguished from that produced by myocardial infarction. If the thoracic aorta is involved, the pain may be referred to the precordial, interscapular, lumbar, or epigastric region. If the abdominal aorta is involved, the pain is usually referred to the lumbar, pelvic, or umbilical regions.

29

CASE

patient did not have a history of diabetes. The hematocrit was 22% (normal, 35 to 47%). The prothrombin time was slightly extended, and the partial thromboplastin time was within normal limits. The patient was immediately sent to the operating room, but she died on the operating table while attempts were made to close the ruptured aortic aneurysm.[5]

At autopsy, the peritoneal cavity was found to be filled with 800 ml of bloody fluid and 300 g of blood clot. There was also considerable edema and hemorrhage into the retroperitoneum. A dissecting aneurysm began just below the graft from previous surgery and extended downward posteriorly to completely surround the common iliac arteries. The abdominal portion of the aneurysm was completely ruptured in its distal 8 cm.[6] The left renal artery ostium was in the posterior false lumen and was 75% occluded. The anterior true lumen was severely narrowed and was calcified

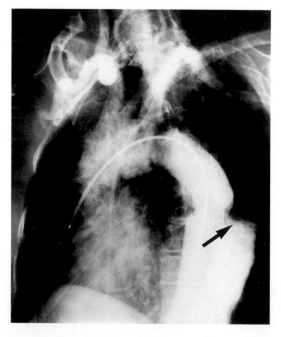

Fig. 5-1. Aortography shows an abrupt change in the apparent diameter of the descending aorta (arrow). This change is the result of extravasation of blood into the fibrous tissue surrounding the aorta.

DISCUSSION

Rupture of an aneurysm is a true medical emergency since the patient can rapidly exsanguinate and die in minutes. Usually, there is a period of pain which precedes the actual rupture of the vessel and during which surgical intervention may be possible. A dropping blood pressure is a sign that significant hemorrhage has occurred and will probably continue.

4. Normal peripheral pulses are rated 2+; absent pulses are rated 0. The Doppler technique uses the echo produced by sound waves to estimate peripheral pulses. The technique is useful when peripheral pulses are difficult to palpate. Peripheral pulses are often asymmetrically reduced in patients with aortic aneurysm. Flow to some arteries may be diminished as a result of occlusive atherosclerosis, thrombus, or pressure from the aneurysm pressing the vessel closed. The distribution of the weakened peripheral pulses, or recent changes in pulses, may suggest the location and extent of the aneurysm.

5. A pulsatile midline mass is practically pathognomonic for an abdominal aortic aneurysm. However, it is sometimes not found, particularly in obese patients. Thoracic aneurysms and aneurysms of the branches of the abdominal aorta are not easily found on physical examination. Diabetic patients tend to develop severe atherosclerosis and consequently have a higher incidence of abdominal aneurysms. Low hematocrit is another indicator of hemorrhage. The hematocrit decreases after hemorrhage as a result of a shift in fluid from extravascular to vascular spaces. Near-normal clotting times indicate that the patient has not developed a bleeding diathesis. This patient's death on the operating table was due to hemorrhage rather than any surgical error.

6. Since total blood volume is approximately 4 L, the quantity of bloody fluid and clot is consistent with substantial hemorrhage. Dissection of the aorta often extends into one or both common iliac arteries. Once an aneurysm begins to rupture, the high blood flow through the break rapidly tears an increasingly larger hole.

7. The occlusion of the left renal artery accounts for the decreased renal function observed clinically. Blood supply to the entire gastrointestinal tract was also impaired, since celiac, superior mesenteric, and inferior mesenteric arteries were all heavily involved with atherosclerosis. Narrowing of the common iliac arteries

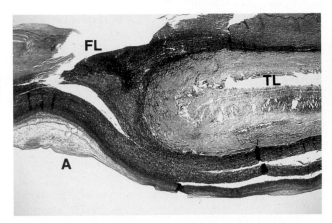

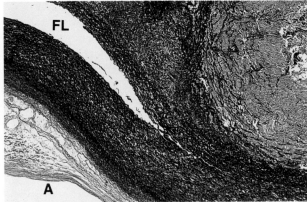

Fig. 5-2. Longitudinal section through an aortic aneurysm (low power photomicrograph, elastic tissue stain). Elastin fibers stain black; muscle stains reddish brown. The adventitia (A) is at the bottom. A portion of the true lumen (TL) is visible to the right. A false lumen (FL) has split the elastic fibers in the aortic wall.

Fig. 5-3. Aortic aneurysm, detail of Fig. 5-1 (high power photomicrograph, Verhoeff stain). In many areas, the elastic fibers are disrupted and are no longer arranged in tightly organized, parallel bundles. This disruption is associated with increased mucopolysaccharide and is characteristic of cystic medial necrosis.

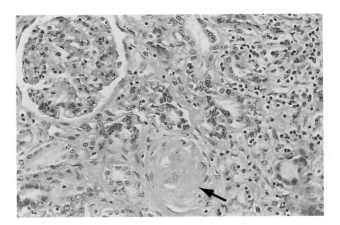

Fig. 5-4. Kidney (high power photomicrograph, hematoxylin and eosin). A lymphocytic infiltration of the renal interstitium is present on the right. A circular area of sclerosis (arrow) may be either a section through the top of a sclerosed glomerulus or a sclerosed blood vessel. The glomerulus present in the upper left corner appears more normal.

CASE

with fractures in the wall. The celiac axis and superior mesenteric artery showed moderate atherosclerosis. The common iliac arteries were severely calcified and narrowed. The ostium of the inferior mesenteric artery could not be identified.[7]

On microscopic examination, the aorta showed increased mucopolysaccharides with extensive atherosclerosis of both false and true lumens (Figs. 5-2 and 5-3). Changes related to diminished renal function included focal sclerosis of glomeruli and periglomerular sclerosis (Fig. 5-4). Also present was atrophy of the renal parenchyma with interstitial fibrosis and mononuclear infiltrates.[8]

DISCUSSION

would have potentially impaired perfusion of pelvic organs and legs. Fractures in calcified plaques may have increased the probability of rupture of the remaining thin wall of the aneurysm.

8. The patient's aneurysm is somewhat unusual in that it appears to be related to two disease processes. The aneurysm was originally a dissecting aneurysm that started in the thoracic aorta. As such, it might have been due to a process such as cystic medial necrosis. The presence of increased mucopolysaccharides suggests that this process was still occurring. Although such aneurysms can extend into the abdominal cavity, they are usually associated with a pure dissection forming a double lumen. Little aneurysmal dilation usually occurs. In this patient, atherosclerosis, also capable of causing abdominal aneurysm, was present to a substantial degree. The atrophy of the renal parenchyma with fibrosis and mononuclear infiltrate may have been secondary to chronically poor renal perfusion. The reason for this patient's focal glomerular and periglomerular sclerosis is unclear.

Aortic Aneurysm

Hypertension in the presence of extensive atherosclerotic involvement of the abdominal aorta can produce a fusiform aneurysm. The aneursym often starts below the renal arteries and may extend into the iliac arteries. This type of aneurysm occurs most frequently in elderly male patients. It can be complicated by thrombosis, emboli to the legs, and fatal bleeding into the peritoneal or retroperitoneal spaces.

Tertiary syphilis, by destruction of elastic tissue in the vessel wall, can cause aneurysms of a variety of shapes that characteristically involve the ascending and transverse portions of the aortic arch. They may extend distally to the diaphragm and proximally to the aortic valve. Complications include fatal hemorrhage and dilation of the aortic valve, producing aortic incompetence. Since the thoracic cavity is a confined space, aneurysms of the arch of the aorta may also produce pressure effects on adjacent structures. Pressure on the recurrent laryngeal nerve may cause persistent cough. Pressure on the vertebrae, sternum, and ribs causes erosion with

pain. The esophagus may be pressed shut, causing difficulty in swallowing. Airways may similarly be pressed completely or partially shut, causing respiratory difficulty.

Cystic medial necrosis is the most common cause of dissecting aneurysms. Focal loss of elastic and muscle fibers in the media produces weakened spaces within the vessel wall that are planes along which dissection can occur. These aneurysms may cut off the blood supply to major aortic branches as the dissection extends.

Questions

1. How do aortic aneurysms develop? What factors can predispose to development of an aortic aneurysm? Which vessels can be affected by a dissecting aortic aneurysm? Describe some of the clinical manifestations that can be produced as abdominal branches of the aorta are affected by the dissection.

2. How was this patient's aortic aneurysm initially treated? What was observed four years after the initial surgical repair of the aneurysm? Why was a second surgical repair not attempted at that time?
3. Why was this patient readmitted to a hospital eight years after her initial surgical repair? What were her symptoms and physical findings? What did laboratory studies show? What happened during her second surgery? What was found at autopsy?

Selected Reading

Bandyk DF: Preoperative imaging of aortic aneurysms. Conventional and digital subtraction angiography, computed tomography scanning, and magnetic resonance imaging. Surg Clin North Am 69:721–735, 1989.

Eagle KA, de Sanctis RW: Aortic dissection. Curr Probl Cardiol 14:225–278, 1989.

6 SEPTICEMIA IN A PATIENT WITH RHEUMATIC HEART DISEASE

Key Words | rheumatic heart disease, mitral stenosis, tricuspid insufficiency, sepsis

CASE

An elderly woman had had rheumatic fever as an 8-year-old child. Although the patient had suffered limitation in her physical activities throughout her life, she had not sought medical help until she was 63. At that time, the patient had decreased exercise tolerance, weight gain, and pedal edema.[1] Right heart catheterization studies showed right atrial pressure of 48 mmHg (normal, <8 mmHg), pulmonary artery pressure of 67/39 mmHg (normal, ca. 25/10 mmHg), pulmonary capillary wedge pressure of 26 mmHg (normal, <8 mmHg), and normal cardiac output. Studies of the left side of the heart showed a mitral valve gradient of 8 mmHg and a normal gradient across the aortic valve.[2] Arterial blood gases on 2 L/min of O_2 per nasal cannula were pH 7.43 (normal, pH 7.38 to 7.44), PCO_2 46 mmHg (normal, 35 to 45 mmHg), and PO_2 63 mmHg (normal, 80 to 100 mmHg).[3]

The diameter of the tricuspid valve was surgically reduced by tricuspid valvuloplasty. The mitral valve was replaced with an artificial valve (Fig. 6-1 and 6-2). Postoperative respiratory distress, thought to be due to pulmonary emboli, was treated with steroids. The patient was released to a

DISCUSSION

1. This patient might have presented in childhood with a severe ("strep") sore throat that progressed to acute rheumatic fever. A surprising number of people with chronic diseases, particularly diseases whose symptoms develop insidiously, do not consult physicians until very late in the clinical course. Decreased exercise tolerance, weight gain, and pedal edema suggest that right-sided heart failure with systemic edema has developed.

2. Markedly increased right atrial pressure suggests an incompetent tricuspid valve, which permits transmission of right ventricular pressures to the right atrium. Increased pulmonary wedge pressures suggest increased left atrial pressures secondary to processes such as left ventricular failure or mitral stenosis. Increased pulmonary wedge pressures can lead to increased pulmonary artery pressures since flow through the lungs is impeded. Normal cardiac output indicates that impaired perfusion due to congestive heart failure or severely stenosed valves has not yet developed. The mitral valve gradient is the pressure difference between the left atrium and left ventricle when the valve is open; it should be near 0 mmHg. A larger gradient demonstrates stenosis of the mitral valve.

3. Slightly increased arterial carbon dioxide tension and

35

CASE

nursing home. Approximately ten weeks after surgery, she was readmitted with dyspnea and tachycardia. Decreased breath sounds were present at the right base.[4] The jugular veins were distended at the angle of the jaw. The heart rate was 138/min and was described as irregularly irregular. A right ventricular heave was present. Electrocardiogram studies showed no acute changes but did show atrial fibrillation with a rate of ventricular contraction of 120 to 130/min (normal 60 to 100/min).[5] The leukocyte count was 13,500 (normal, 4,500 to 11,000). An incidental finding was a clean, open wound on the patient's right upper thigh, which appeared to be a surgically opened abscess. No history was noted in the chart about this wound, which may have been opened at the nursing home. Arterial blood gases on room air were pH 7.55, PCO_2 32 mmHg, and PO_2 46 mmHg. On 2 L/min of O_2, they were pH 7.53, 35 mmHg, and 60 mmHg.[6]

Severe pulmonary hypertension had been a previous diagnosis. Cor pulmonale was thought to have worsened, with possible volume depletion causing a low left-sided filling pressure. The next day, the patient was admitted to a critical care unit, where a Doppler sonogram showed a hypokinetic right ventricle with a grossly normal left ventricle.

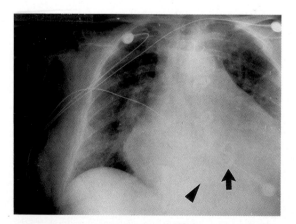

Fig. 6-1. Chest radiograph shows a massively enlarged heart. A radiopaque ring reinforces the tricuspid valve (arrowhead); the mitral valve has been replaced with an artificial valve (arrow). The two superior radiopaque structures are bands reinforcing the sternal closure.

DISCUSSION

decreased arterial oxygen tension, despite increased oxygen concentrations in inspired air, suggest that significant pulmonary edema has impaired blood oxygenation. The patient's cardiac pathophysiology at the time of surgery can be interpreted as being probably due the following sequence of events. The rheumatic fever many years previously damaged the mitral valve. Over the years, mitral stenosis developed. The stenosis caused left atrial pressures to increase, which in turn caused pulmonary capillary and then pulmonary artery pressures to increase. The increased pulmonary artery pressures caused increased pressure and dilation of the right ventricle. Dilation of the right ventricle stretched the tricuspid orifice, causing it to be incompetent. Finally, the incompetent tricuspid valve caused right atrial pressures to increase.

4. Valvuloplasty involves partially suturing valve leaflets to reduce the lumen of an incompetent valve. Replacement of a valve with an artificial valve is indicated when the original valve has been so badly damaged that repair is not feasible. Risk factors for pulmonary embolism in this patient include the surgical manipulation of the heart, right cardiac chamber dilation, and the venous stasis associated with both bed rest and prolonged surgical procedures. After surgery, the patient did reasonably well for a few months and then had an abrupt progressive illness that led to her death within a few days. Dyspnea, tachycardia, and decreased breath sounds may be due to either primary pulmonary problems, such as pneumonia, or secondary to primary cardiac disease, such as congestive heart failure with pulmonary edema.

5. The jugular venous distension suggests that increased right atrial filling pressures were present. The right ventricular heave was probably related to right ventricular hypertrophy. The phrase "irregularly irregular heart rate" denotes periods of reasonably regular heart rate interspersed with periods of very irregular heart rate. This pattern is characteristic of atrial fibrillation. Atrial fibrillation predisposes to pulmonary and systemic emboli since blood clots can form in the dilated atria and then later embolize.

6. The patient's increased leukocyte count suggests that she might have an infection, possibly a pneumonia because of the decreased breath sounds. It is not uncommon for elderly patients transferred from a nursing home to be admitted with a poorly documented

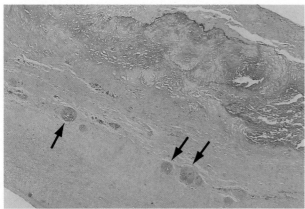

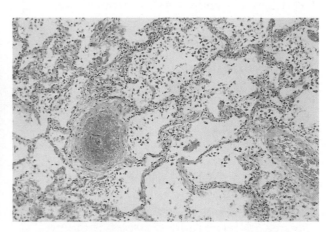

Fig. 6-2. Mitral valve damaged by rheumatic heart disease (low power photomicrograph, hematoxylin and eosin, from another case). Calcification of this markedly thickened and fibrotic mitral valve is visible as fine blue lines in the upper right quadrant. Vascularization (*arrows*) of the normally avascular mitral valve is also seen. These changes are typical of those seen years after rheumatic heart disease has damaged a mitral valve.

Fig. 6-3. Pneumonia (high power photomicrograph, hematoxylin and eosin). A mild, patchy consolidative process is present that was thought to be due to viral infection. This level of pneumonia was not considered sufficient to cause the patient's death. Note the slight thickening of alveolar septae and perivascular fibrosis consistent with pulmonary hypertension.

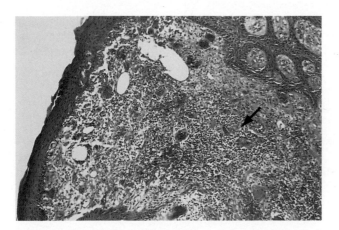

Fig. 6-4. Subcutaneous abscess (low power photomicrograph, hematoxylin and eosin, from another case). A subcutaneous infiltration with neutrophils (*arrow*) is accompanied by tissue necrosis and hemorrhage. Large subcutaneous abscesses can extend completely through the subcutaneous fat and connective tissue and into the underlying muscle.

CASE

Rapid closure indicated a low stroke volume. Later that day, there was evidence of embolization with a cold, pulseless, cyanotic right arm. The patient progressed to coma, had a respiratory arrest with bradycardia, and then died.[7]

At autopsy, the lungs showed only minimal evidence of pulmonary hypertension. Mild chronic obstructive lung disease and a patchy consolidative process that was probably viral in origin were also present (Fig. 6-3). The heart showed mitral valve replacement, tricuspid valvuloplasty, and cardiomegaly with bilateral atrial enlargement and biventricular hypertrophy. None of these pulmonary or cardiovascular problems appeared sufficiently severe to explain the patient's death. However, there was also evidence of sepsis and disseminated intravascular coagulation: multiple fibrin clots and bleeding were present in many tissues, and the kidney contained numerous small, recent infarcts. The spleen and liver showed polymorphonuclear infiltrates, commonly associated with sepsis. The surgically opened abscess appeared to be the source of the infection (Fig. 6-4). Autopsy blood cultures were positive for *Escherichia coli* and *Klebsiella pneumoniae*.[8]

DISCUSSION

history. Furthermore, these patients may be unable to clearly describe why certain treatments were performed. The pneumonia was not sufficiently severe to cause dangerous levels in arterial blood gases while the patient was on nasal O_2.

7. Throughout the day following readmission, the right-sided heart difficulties progressed to right cardiac failure as indicated by the hypokinetic right ventricle and low stroke volume identified by Doppler ultrasonography. The patient then became comatose and died of respiratory and cardiac arrest.

8. Unfortunately, it is not always clear why a patient, with an apparently minor illness, does very poorly. In this case, evidence of an unsuspected bacterial sepsis was found at autopsy. Since the sepsis was unsuspected, the patient was never treated with antibiotics. However, even if the sepsis had been recognized, it is not clear that the final outcome would have been different. There is at present no definitive therapy for bacterial endotoxin-induced shock, and appropriate measures would have been general supportive measures similar to what she received anyway. The source of the bacteremia was apparently a surgically corrected abscess on her thigh, perhaps due to a bedsore, that was not included in her history and was considered to be only an incidental finding during the physical examination.

Rheumatic Heart Disease

Rheumatic fever is an acute disease that usually presents in childhood. It occurs after infection by group A beta-hemolytic streptococci in throat or skin lesions, but appears to more closely resemble an autoimmune process than an infection. The disease that develops appears to be due to cross-reactivity between streptococcal antigens and host antigens. Major manifestations of acute rheumatic fever include a migratory arthritis involving large joints; a pancarditis that may lead to left ventricular failure, pericarditis, or involvement of the heart valves; a chorea that presents with constant, purposeless muscular activity; painless and freely movable subcutaneous nodules; and a distinctive rash known as erythema marginatum that begins as reddish macules

that rapidly expand into large confluent circles. Not all manifestations are present in each patient. Most symptoms resolve without permanent sequelae over a period of weeks to a few months. However, endocarditis can develop and can lead to progressive involvement of the valves in the heart; this may, usually over many years, seriously compromise cardiac performance.

Although the full-blown presentation of acute rheumatic fever can be very dramatic, it appears clear that much milder, and possibly even subclinical, forms of the disease exist and may damage the heart. Thus, many patients who later develop rheumatic valvular disease may have either a very remote history of rheumatic fever or even no known history. In the acute stage, rheumatic fever damages a valve by causing an inflammatory reaction characterized predominantly by edema, although fibrinoid necrosis of connective tissues may also occur. The swollen valve is then repeatedly traumatized during valve closure; this leads to the formation of verrucous fibrin deposits at the tips of the leaflets. Valves that sustain the highest pressures (mitral, aortic, and tricuspid) are the most vulnerable. Eventually, over many years, the repeated injuries and repairs lead to deformation of the valve. A valve damaged by disease can become either stenotic, when scar tissue narrows the valve orifice, or incompetent, when valve leaflets are so torn or distorted by disease that they no longer can completely occlude the valvular lumen.

Questions

1. What types of cardiac disease can rheumatic fever produce? At what age did this patient have rheumatic fever? At what age did she require medical attention for her rheumatic heart disease? What symptoms did she experience at that time? What did laboratory studies show?

2. What was the pathophysiology of this patient's mitral and tricuspid valvular disease? Which of her signs, symptoms, and laboratory findings were related to each of these valves? How was her valvular disease treated?

3. Why was this patient readmitted ten weeks after surgery? Discuss her physical examination and laboratory studies at the time of readmission. What medical problems was she thought to have? How did she die? What was found at autopsy?

Selected Reading

Assey ME, Spann JF Jr: Indications for heart valve replacement. Clin Cardiol 13:81–88, 1990.

Douglas PS: Rheumatic heart disease and other valvular disorders in women. Cardiovasc Clin 19:259–269, 1989.

7 ARRHYTHMIAS COMPLICATING CONGESTIVE HEART FAILURE

Key Words | atherosclerosis, myocardial infarction, congestive heart failure

CASE

A 75-year-old man had a long history of atherosclerotic heart disease. His first myocardial infarction had occurred five years previously. He had recovered without complication from this first infarction and was reasonably well for four years. He then had a second myocardial infarction, after which he developed congestive heart failure with pedal edema. A chest radiograph showed an enlarged cardiac profile (Fig. 7-1). Immediately after the second infarction, his heart rate and rhythm were appropriate with no evidence of arrhythmia.[1] The patient recovered well enough to be sent home after therapy with salt restriction, digoxin, and furosemide. He was readmitted several months later for increasingly severe congestive heart failure.[2] Electrocardiographic studies showed junctional rhythm with a left bundle branch block. The patient also had many premature ventricular contractions. Digoxin and furosemide dosages were increased, with better control of the congestive heart failure. Quinidine was added to treat the arrhythmia.[3]

The patient was released and was fairly well for the next six months. He then had an episode of syncope with nausea and vomiting. His wife noted

DISCUSSION

1. Hypertrophy of remaining myocardial fibers can sometimes restore the heart's ability to pump blood at normal pressure and volume. The risk of developing permanent sequelae increases with each subsequent heart attack. Congestive heart failure develops when the heart no longer meets the body's perfusion requirements. Arrhythmias develop when myocardial infarction damages the pacemakers and/or the conducting system of the heart. The patient's pedal edema indicated that right ventricular failure was present. Left-sided heart failure may also have been present, producing pulmonary edema, but was not specifically indicated at this stage of the patient's history.

2. Diuretics, such as furosemide, improve cardiac function by reducing edema and lowering the blood volume. Agents that improve cardiac contractility, such as digoxin, improve the heart's ability to pump.

3. Development of a junctional rhythm indicated that the sinoatrial node was no longer performing adequately. The bundle branch block indicated that the cardiac conduction system was also impaired. The conducting system and sinoatrial node can be damaged by both myocardial infarction and cardiac hypertrophy. Premature ventricular contractions are contractions initiated by an ectopic pacemaker that occur

41

CASE

that he was cyanotic and perspired excessively. He was brought by medics to a hospital, where he was found to be in sustained ventricular tachycardia. The tachycardia was initially corrected with intravenous lidocaine. However, it recurred repeatedly, and the patient was treated with multiple cardioversions and a variety of antiarrhythmic agents. He was transferred to an intensive care unit, where he was placed on a ventilator.[4]

Physical examination showed an unresponsive man who was hypotensive. The pulse was 110/min (normal, 60 to 100 min). The pupils were fixed and dilated. The neck was supple, with prominent jugular venous distension. Diffuse rales were detected in the lungs. The heart was inaudible. After transfer to the intensive care unit, the patient required both dopamine and dobutamine for a systolic blood pressure of 90 to 100 mmHg.[5] He also required an inspired oxygen fraction of 100% with 15-cm positive end-expiratory pressure to maintain a PO_2 of 64 mmHg (normal, 80 to 100 mmHg). The cardiac rhythm remained stable with a wide complex junctional rhythm. The pupils continued to be fixed and dilated after treatment, and the patient assumed the decerebrate posture in response to sternal pressure. Six hours later the patient went into intractable ventricular tachycardia and died. Permission for autopsy was restricted to the thorax only.[6]

The patient was found at autopsy to have severe triple vessel coronary artery atherosclerosis (Fig. 7-2). Evidence of extensive old myocardial infarction was present in anterior, posterior, and septal regions of the ventricles. Fibrosis was grossly apparent in at least 30% of the myocardium. There were no areas sectioned that showed acute myocardial infarction. Also present was severe cardiomegaly with four-chamber dilation and biventricular hypertrophy.[7] Examination of the lungs demonstrated severe longstanding congestion and confirmed the clinical evidence of previous pulmonary edema. Hemosiderin-laden macrophages and hemorrhage were also present. There was also evidence of moderate pulmonary hypertension (Fig. 7-3). The cause of death was considered to be ischemic cardiomyopathy.[8]

DISCUSSION

before the normal electrical signal reaches the ventricles. They occur more commonly when a bundle branch block impairs conduction of the normal electrical signal. Premature ventricular contractions have little clinical significance when they occur rarely. Frequent premature ventricular contractions may initiate ventricular tachycardia.

4. The description of the patient's episode of syncope is a classic description of sudden onset of life-threatening ventricular tachycardia. Many of the symptoms experienced are related to hypotension, since the heart's ability to pump effectively may be badly compromised by inadequate chamber filling times. Massive autonomic outflow also contributes to the symptoms. Many drugs have antiarrhythmic activity. Although some information is available about the effectiveness of particular drugs in various arrhythmias, it is often necessary to try many drugs before a patient's arrhythmia can be adequately controlled. Sometimes, damage to the heart continues to progress to the point that no drug can be found to control the arrhythmia. Many arrhythmias are self-sustaining once started. Massive electrical stimulation of the heart, known as cardioversion, may then be necessary. Antiarrhythmic medications are usually given after cardioversion to try to prevent reinitiation of the arrhythmia.

5. Fixed and dilated pupils suggest severe cerebral cortical damage. Prominent jugular venous distension indicates severe right-sided heart failure. The fact that the heart was inaudible suggests that it was pumping so weakly that normal cardiac sounds were no longer produced. Diffuse rales indicate pulmonary edema and left-sided heart failure. Dopamine and dobutamine both improve cardiac contractility but have opposing effects on peripheral vasculature. Their joint use enhances contractility while minimizing the effects on blood vessels.

6. The patient's blood gas studies reflect the limitations on oxygen diffusion in his edematous lungs. The decerebrate posture is assumed either spontaneously or in response to external stimuli and indicates damage, usually irreversible, to the brainstem. The entire body becomes stiff, and the arms assume a characteristic position close to the side of the body with the forearms pronated and the fingers and wrists flexed.

7. Ischemic damage is less easily limited by the develop-

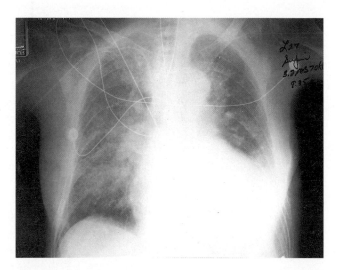

Fig. 7-1. Chest radiograph showing enlarged cardiac profile.

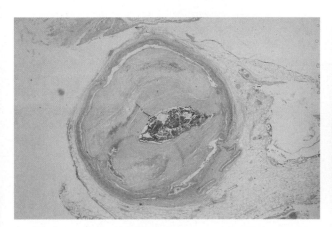

Fig. 7-2. Coronary atherosclerosis (low power photomicrograph, hematoxylin and eosin). The coronary artery shows severe atherosclerosis with marked narrowing of the vessel lumen. This degree of narrowing limits the blood flow to the cardiac muscle.

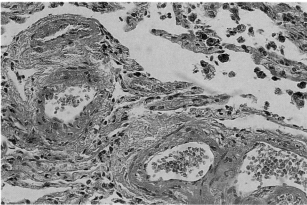

Fig. 7-3. Pulmonary hypertension (high power photomicrograph, hematoxylin and eosin). Several vessel profiles are present in this field. These profiles are probably sections through a single tortuous arteriole. The vessel wall shows thickening of the smooth muscle, consistent with moderate pulmonary hypertension. The adjacent alveoli contain darkly staining, hemosiderin-laden macrophages. Such macrophages indicate the presence of previous intra-alveolar hemorrhage.

DISCUSSION

ment of collateral circulation when atherosclerosis seriously involves several coronary arteries. If a patient survives a myocardial infarction for longer than several months, the necrotic tissue is replaced by fibrosis. Given the extent of involvement of the myocardium by fibrosis, it is not surprising that this patient developed intractable arrhythmias. Biventricular hypertrophy may have represented an attempt by the remaining functioning myocardium to compensate by hypertrophy for the tissue loss to infarction. Alternatively, chronic hypertension is associated with ventricular hypertrophy. Chamber dilation occurs when portions of the cardiac wall do not contract effectively and consequently are slowly stretched during systole.

8. Hemosiderin-laden macrophages are evidence of previous intra-alveolar hemorrhage, which can occur with damage by hypertension or congestion to the alveolar capillary bed. Chronic pulmonary congestion produces dilated alveolar capillaries. The alveolar septa may become widened by both these capillaries and interstitial edema. Pulmonary hypertension is associated microscopically with increased thickness of arterial walls. The arteries in the lung parenchyma eventually resemble systemic arteries more closely than the normal thin-walled branches of the pulmonary artery system.

Heart Failure

Heart failure can involve either or both ventricles; it typically produces diminished cardiac output and fatigue. When the right ventricle fails, elevated back pressure in systemic veins manifests clinically as increased jugular venous pressure, peripheral edema, ascites, and an enlarged, tender liver. When the left ventricle fails, pulmonary venous and capillary pressures rise, leading to pulmonary edema as fluid leaks into the pulmonary interstitium and alveoli. Failure of both ventricles produces a combined picture. Right ventricular failure is usually caused by increased pulmonary arterial pressure. Such increased pressure may be caused by either lung disease, leading to cor pulmonale, or left ventricular failure. Right ventricular failure also occurs in congenital heart disease or as a result of acquired lesions of

the tricuspid or pulmonary valve. Left ventricular failure can be caused by problems directly affecting cardiac muscle such as ischemic heart disease, myocarditis, infiltrations of the heart, and cardiomyopathies. Alternatively, it can occur secondary to other cardiac or circulatory problems such as cardiac arrhythmias, valvular disease involving the mitral or aortic valves, systemic hypertension, severe anemia, and large arteriovenous shunts. In some of these conditions, cardiac output may be greater than normal, but still less than is needed for adequate oxygenation of tissues.

Questions

1. What factors can predispose a patient for myocardial infarction? How many myocardial infarctions did

this patient have? What are the potential complications of a myocardial infarction? At what point did this patient develop an arrhythmia? What measures were initially used to treat this patient's arrhythmia and worsening congestive heart failure?

2. What were the patient's presenting complaints at his final admission? What problem was diagnosed? Why is sustained ventricular tachycardia dangerous? What measures were used to treat his arrhythmias during his final admission? How successful were these measures?

3. What problem did this patient develop immediately after transfer to the university hospital? Why did this problem complicate the control of his arrhythmias? How did the patient die? What was found at autopsy?

Selected Reading

Klitzner TS, Friedman WF: Cardiac arrhythmias: the role of pharmacologic intervention. Cardiol Clin 7:299–318, 1989.

Parmley WW: Pathophysiology and current therapy of congestive heart failure. J Am Coll Cardiol 13:771–785, 1989.

8 PERIPARTUM CONGESTIVE CARDIOMYOPATHY

Key Words | pregnancy, cardiomyopathy, congestive heart failure

CASE

A 26-year-old woman had delivered her most recent child ten days previously. The patient was morbidly obese. The obstetric history included nine spontaneous vaginal deliveries, several therapeutic abortions, and several spontaneous abortions. The patient had developed shortness of breath during the third trimester of the most recent pregnancy.[1] An echocardiogram taken at that time revealed massive dilation of all four chambers with mitral regurgitation and tricuspid regurgitation.[2] The patient was treated with the potent loop diuretic bumetanide, the cardiac stimulant digoxin, and potassium supplement. She had an uneventful delivery of a 3 lb, 3 oz (1400 kg) baby by normal spontaneous vaginal delivery. There were no peripartum complications. The patient was discharged and went home, spending most of the intervening time in bed. When she climbed stairs, she experienced a sharp pain in the left chest radiating to the back. She also reported increasing shortness of breath and small amounts of blood-tinged sputum. She continued to have orthopnea and slept in a sitting position. There was no history of fever or chills or change in the lochia.[3]

The patient's father had died of a sudden cardiac arrest at age 49 with a history of type II diabetes mellitus. Two sisters have leg swelling and shortness of breath but have never seen a doctor

DISCUSSION

1. The patient's age and obstetric history suggest that inadequate postpartum recovery may have complicated some pregnancies. Mild shortness of breath can occur in normal pregnancies simply as a result of impairment of abdominal breathing by the bulk of the uterus. More serious shortness of breath suggests that a pathological process such as pneumonia or pulmonary edema may be present.

2. The cardiac condition had probably been developing during earlier pregnancies, but was not apparent until the final pregnancy. Massive dilation of the heart suggests that it was not contracting effectively. Such dilation can impair the competence of cardiac valves and produce regurgitation. The onset of regurgitation may have triggered the apparently sudden onset of symptoms.

3. The patient's congestive heart failure appeared to be well controlled by medication since the delivery was uneventful and she recovered well enough to be sent home. Sharp pain on climbing stairs was suggestive of angina. Persistent congestive heart failure is suggested by the patient's orthopnea and habit of sleeping in a sitting position. Infection might have been suggested by fevers, chills, or changes in vaginal secretions, known in the postpartum period as lochia.

4. Some cases of peripartum congestive cardiomyopathy appear to begin with subclinical damage that may have a familial basis. The children may have also been separated from each other, since a single foster

CASE

to assess whether these symptoms are cardiac in origin. The patient did not smoke or consume alcohol. After her admission, her children were placed in foster homes with the exception of the new baby, who remained at the hospital.[4]

Physical examination revealed a pulse of 120/min (normal, 60 to 100/min), blood pressure of 110/60 mmHg (normal, 100 to 140/60 to 90 mmHg), respiratory rate of 24/min (normal, 6 to 20/min), and temperature of 37.2°C (normal, 37.0°C). The neck showed jugular venous pulse at the angle of the jaws. Bilateral rales and occasional expiratory wheezes were present. Cardiac examination revealed two distinct systolic ejection murmurs heard best respectively at the apex and over the aortic area. There were separate right and left ventricular impulses. The liver was enlarged on palpation. Extremities showed pitting edema without clubbing or cyanosis.[5]

The patient was suspected of having congestive heart failure secondary to cardiomyopathy. She was treated aggressively with bed rest, diuretics, inotropic support, and fluid and sodium restriction. Pulmonary embolus was also suspected and was confirmed by a pulmonary angiogram. Anticoagulants were added to the therapeutic regimen. The patient remained clinically stable and was losing weight. She experienced vaginal bleeding, which was thought to be due to heparinization. The anticoagulant was changed to the milder oral anticoagulant warfarin.[6] After two weeks, the patient was feeling better but clinically remained the same except for loss of 7 lb (3 kg) of body weight. Bilateral rales and peripheral edema continued to be present. An echocardiogram done one week after admission revealed four-chamber enlargement with moderate pericardial effusion. The patient had two episodes of hemoptysis five days later. Three weeks after admission, she was found apneic and pulseless and was pronounced dead.[7]

At autopsy, a huge heart was noted which showed dilation of all chambers and hypertrophy of both ventricles. Pericardial effusion (500 ml) was present (Fig. 8-1). Multiple pulmonary emboli were present in the pulmonary arteries of both lungs. The lungs were heavy and had multiple wedge-shaped firm areas of infarct and hemor-

DISCUSSION

home was probably not found. Good medical care sometimes involves considering non-medical implications of serious illness for both the patient and family.

5. Both pulse and respirations were rapid. Increased jugular venous pressure suggests right-sided heart failure. Rales suggest pulmonary edema, probably the result of left-sided heart failure. The ejection murmurs were probably related to previously documented valvular insufficiency. Separate right and left ventricular impulses suggest right ventricular hypertrophy. The enlarged liver was probably the result of hepatic congestion secondary to increased central venous pressures. Pitting edema indicates right-sided heart failure.

6. Pulmonary emboli tend to occur in patients confined to bed for prolonged periods. Pulmonary emboli can exacerbate respiratory difficulties that were initially due to pulmonary edema. Careful management may be required in patients at risk for both hemorrhage and embolus formation.

7. The persistence of pulmonary and cardiac findings indicated that the patient's disease was not resolving. Pericardial effusion may be a dangerous complication, since the heart's ability to fill during diastole may be compromised. Pulmonary embolus can cause hemoptysis. It is a relatively common cause of acute exacerbation of symptoms related to congestive heart failure.

8. Massive pericardial effusion may have contributed to the patient's cardiac dysfunction. Pulmonary infarction can occur secondary to embolus. Because of the distributions of the pulmonary circulations, pulmonary infarcts are characteristically wedge-shaped and "point" toward the embolus.

9. Tracheobronchitis is a common complication caused by abrasion of the upper airways during intubation. Congestion in the spleen and liver was probably initially the result of right-sided heart failure. Later, the thrombus in the inferior vena cava may have impaired drainage through the hepatic veins.

10. Many cardiomyopathies are still poorly understood, in part because the findings are often nonspecific. Dilated, poorly contracting atria and ventricles can form a surface for thrombosis. Pieces of thrombi may then break off and embolize to either the pulmonary or systemic circulation. Increased ground substance is a common nonspecific finding in severe regurgitation.

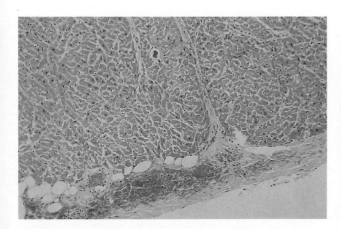

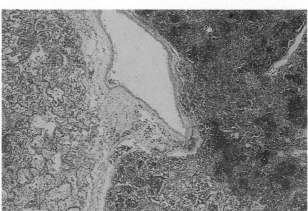

Fig. 8-1. Pericardial hemorrhage (low power photomicrograph, hematoxylin and eosin). The cardiac muscle fibers *(above)* are somewhat enlarged but otherwise appear near normal. The pericardial surface *(below)* is thickened and contains focal lymphocytic infiltration and hemorrhage. Leakage of fluid through the damaged pericardial surface probably contributed to the patient's prominent pericardial effusion (500 ml) noted at autopsy.

Fig. 8-2. Pulmonary infarction (low power photomicrograph, hematoxylin and eosin). The infarcted lung *(right)* is sharply demarcated from damaged, but still surviving, adjacent lung *(left)*. This sharp demarcation reflects the lobular organization of the blood supply to the lung. The infarcted tlssue is grossly hemorrhagic owing to the double blood supply (branches of the pulmonary and bronchial arteries) to the lung.

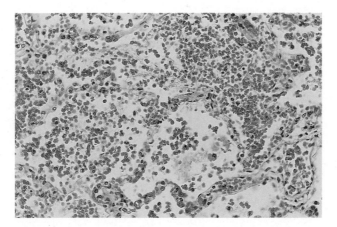

Fig. 8-3. Lung, detail of Fig. 8-2 (high power photomicrograph, hematoxylin and eosin). The alveoli illustrated are from the left side of Fig. 8-2. These alveoli contain hemorrhage, but they still contain viable cells, as indicated by the dark nuclei visible in the alveolar walls.

CASE

rhage (Figs. 8-2 and 8-3).[8] Tracheobronchitis secondary to respiratory therapy was also present. The liver was enlarged, with centrilobular congestion and necrosis. There was also congestive splenomegaly. An inferior vena caval thrombosis was located in the proximal portion of the vessel.[9]

Histologically, the myocardium showed only nonspecific changes of hypertrophic muscle fibers with some nuclear changes. The pulmonary emboli in this patient probably originated from mural thrombi in the right ventricle or from the inferior vena caval clot. The inferior vena caval thrombosis can be considered secondary to catheterization. The left atrium showed increased thickness due to increased ground substance. The cause of death was pulmonary embolism and infarction, with poor left ventricular function and pericardial effusion also contributing.[10]

Cardiomyopathies

The term *cardiomyopathy* is used when a disease process principally involves cardiac myocytes. Excluded are diseases that are the result of processes, such as hypertension, valvular disease, and congenital defects, elsewhere in the heart. Cardiomyopathies are often classified in terms of either clinical manifestations or etiology. Many cases of cardiomyopathy are idiopathic. When the cause has been identified, a variety of etiologies have been found: drugs or toxins; allergic reactions; viral, bacterial, fungal, protozoal, or metazoal infections; metabolic, nutrient deficiency, or storage diseases; connective tissue disorders; infiltrations and granulomas; and neuromuscular diseases. Clinical classes of cardiomyopathy include congestive, restrictive, and hypertrophic cardiomyopathies. Occasionally, cardiomyopathy will have features of intermediate character.

In congestive cardiomyopathies, the myocardium becomes weak and contracts poorly. These cardiomyopathies are characterized by a large, dilated heart with impaired systolic function. There is a tendency to develop congestive heart failure, arrhythmias, and mural thrombi. Examples of cardiomyopathies that produce a congestive pattern include alcoholic cardiomyopathy, peripartum cardiomyopathy, and several muscular dystrophies. In restrictive cardiomyopathy, scarring or myocardial infiltration limits the ability of the ventricles to dilate during diastole. These cardiomyopathies are characterized by decreased cardiac output. Persistently elevated venous pressure produces hepatic congestion, edema, and ascites. Examples of restrictive cardiomyopathies include endomyocardial fibrosis and infiltration of the myocardium by amyloid or hemochromatosis. In hypertrophic cardiomyopathy, the basic defect involves hypertrophy of the cardiac wall. The hypertrophy usually disproportionately involves the left ventricle, often the ventricular septum in particular. Outflow of the aorta may be obstructed. Many patients with hypertrophic cardiomyopathies are asymptomatic. In a few, the only clinical manifestation is sudden death after physical exertion. Dyspnea, angina pectoris, fatigue, and syncope are common in patients who are symptomatic. Most patients with hypertrophic cardiomyopathy have an idiopathic disease that may have a familial predisposition. A few have other diseases such as Friedreich's ataxia.

Questions

1. Describe this patient's obstetric history. What had happened during her most recent pregnancy? How was she treated? Was her delivery or her baby affected by her cardiac problems?
2. Why was the patient readmitted ten days after delivery? What symptoms was she experiencing? What risk factors for cardiac disease did she have? Describe the findings on physical examination.
3. How was the patient treated after admission? What complications did she experience? How did she die? What was found at autopsy? What do you think the consequences of her death were for her family?

Selected Reading

Dunmire SM: Pulmonary embolism. Emerg Med Clin N Am 7:339–354, 1989.
Gianopoulos JG: Cardiac disease in pregnancy. Med Clin N Am 73:639–651, 1989
Parmley WW: Pathophysiology and current therapy of congestive heart failure. J Am Coll Cardiol 13:771–785, 1989.

HEMATOLOGY

9 AMYLOIDOSIS IN A PATIENT WITH MULTIPLE MYELOMA

Key Words | multiple myeloma, amyloidosis, congestive heart failure, nephrotic syndrome

CASE

A 48-year-old woman presented with bilateral carpal tunnel syndrome and underwent bilateral surgical release procedures.[1] Three months later, she developed some shortness of breath with fever. She was thought to have bronchitis and was treated with antibiotics, and the episode resolved. One month later, the symptoms recurred and the patient also noted alopecia and palpable purpura on her fingers.[2] Seven months after her presentation with bilateral carpal tunnel syndrome, she was admitted to a community hospital with a chief complaint of dyspnea on exertion. The physical examination on admission showed jugular venous distention, basilar rales, and pedal edema.[3] The serum total protein was 4.9 g/100 ml (normal, 6.3 to 7.7 g/100 ml) with a serum albumin of 2.3 g/100 ml (normal, 3.5 to 5.5 g/100 ml.) The 24-hour urine total protein was 11.7 g (normal, <150 mg). Creatinine clearance was within normal limits.[4] The results of serological tests for rheumatoid factor, antinuclear antibodies, and anti-DNA antibodies were all negative. A renal sonogram showed no hydronephrosis, but a possible bulge was visible in the superior pole of the right kidney.[5] The results of gingival and rectal biopsies were positive for amyloid. Vigorous diuresis led to a 40-lb weight loss. The patient was transferred to a university hospital for further

DISCUSSION

1. Compression of the median nerve in the carpal tunnel produces weakness of the thenar muscles and paresthesias on the palmar surface of the fingers. The bilateral presence of carpal tunnel syndrome suggests that the underlying process is systemic rather than local.

2. This case illustrates the insidiousness of some diseases. At first glance, the patient's hand symptoms, shortness of breath with fever, hair loss, and purpura appear unrelated. Hair loss is the first indication that the patient may be seriously ill. Palpable purpura suggests focal hemorrhage in the dermis. An early, extensive evaluation of nonspecific symptoms such as these can be expensive, involves risk to the patient, and may actually exclude the diagnosis that later proves to be correct, since all of the findings necessary for a diagnosis may not yet be present.

3. Possible involvement of the patient's cardiovascular system was first indicated by dyspnea on exertion. Jugular venous distention and pedal edema suggest that the patient's right ventricle was failing. Rales suggest pulmonary edema caused by left-sided heart failure. An extensive evaluation was clearly appropriate at this point because of the rapidly progressive cardiac symptoms.

4. Nephrotic syndrome is indicated by the conjunction of significant proteinuria, low serum protein levels, and edema. A normal or near-normal glomerular fil-

55

CASE

evaluation and management. Her admitting diagnoses were amyloidosis with nephrotic syndrome, dehydration, and congestive heart failure.[6]

Laboratory studies showed a slight elevation of serum calcium, normal hematocrit and hemoglobin, and normal platelet and leukocyte counts.[7] Increased interstitial pulmonary marking was noted on a chest radiograph (Fig. 9-1). An echocardiogram revealed an enlarged right ventricle and a hypoplastic left ventricle. A Swan-Ganz catheter study gave results consistent with moderately severe pulmonary hypertension and right-sided heart failure.[8] Quantitative studies of immunoglobulins showed low IgG and IgA concentrations. A biclonal pattern was noted. A bone marrow biopsy revealed a diffuse plasmacytosis. Biopsy specimens from the papules on the patient's finger were positive for amyloid.[9]

The patient was discharged and over the next few weeks experienced increasing shortness of breath. Two weeks before another admission, she stopped taking furosemide. She was readmitted

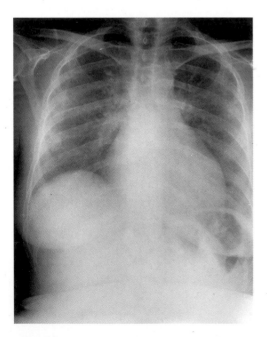

Fig. 9-1. Chest radiograph shows prominent parenchymal markings caused by deposition of amyloid around blood vessels and bronchi.

DISCUSSION

tration rate can coexist with nephrotic syndrome when a small percentage of severely damaged glomeruli leak substantial amounts of protein.

5. Positive serological test results would have suggested diseases with autoimmune components, such as systemic lupus erythematosus. The renal sonogram might have revealed obstruction or stones.

6. Amyloidosis, in which protein fragments are deposited in tissue, is a cause of nephrotic syndrome. Patients with significant edema may have surprisingly large quantities of excess water. Vigorous diuresis will remove this fluid and often improves cardiopulmonary function, but it may be difficult to titrate the diuresis so that as much excess fluid is removed as possible without dehydrating the patient.

7. Renal disease can cause hypercalcemia and, in some patients, osteoporosis and secondary hyperparathyroidism as a result of altered vitamin D metabolism and altered excretion of electrolytes.

8. Increased interstitial pulmonary markings suggest thickened alveolar or bronchiolar walls. Such thickening can be produced by scarring and infiltration by cells or acellular deposits. A hypoplastic left ventricle indicates impaired myocardial contraction, possibly due to infarction or deposition of amyloid in the heart. A Swan-Ganz catheter is a pressure-sensitive device that is inserted sequentially through a large vein, the right atrium, the right ventricle, and the pulmonary artery. Pulmonary hypertension can be demonstrated by pressure measurements taken in the pulmonary artery. The combination of severe pulmonary hypertension and right-sided heart failure is a common cause of right ventricular enlargement.

9. A bone marrow biopsy showing plasmacytosis and an altered electrophoresis pattern suggests multiple myeloma. Multiple myeloma can cause amyloidosis when free lambda light chains and proteins with similar structure are deposited in the patient's tissues. Since a myeloma cell line usually produces a single immunoglobulin, most multiple myeloma patients have only a single clonal spike. The presence of two clonal spikes (biclonal pattern) was unusual and may have indicated the presence of two distinct myeloma cell lines. This may also have contributed to the unusually rapid progression of this patient's amyloidosis. Once the diagnosis of multiple myeloma was made, a number of clinical findings could be reinter-

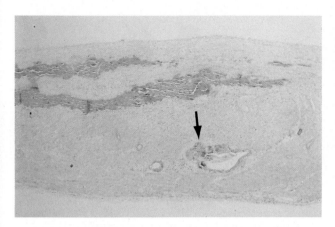

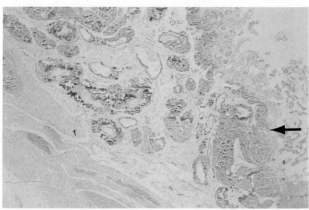

Fig. 9-2. Amyloidosis involving the heart (low power photomicrograph, Congo red). Amyloid stains with Congo red; other tissue elements remain light gray. Most of the amyloid is deposited as a thick band, doubled in places, in the muscle. Some is also deposited around vessel walls *(arrow)*.

Fig. 9-3. Amyloidosis involving the gastrointestinal tract (low power photomicrograph, Congo red). The intestinal muscle is on the lower left; the mucosal surface is on the upper right. A heavy band of amyloid is deposited below the mucosa *(arrow)*. Additional amyloid is deposited around blood vessels in the submucosa. A smaller amount of amyloid has infiltrated some muscle bundles. Despite this extensive amyloidosis, the patient did not complain of prominent gastrointestinal symptoms.

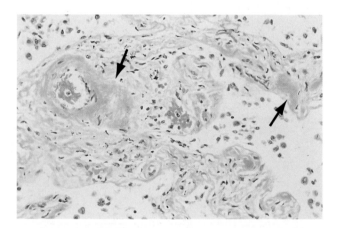

Fig. 9-4. Amyloidosis in the lung (high power photomicrograph, hematoxylin and eosin). An unusual feature of this case was the prominent deposition of amyloid in the lungs. Slides stained with hematoxylin and eosin show eosinophilic deposits *(arrows)* in the alveolar walls and around blood vessels. These eosinophilic deposits are definitively identified as amyloid by staining similar tissue sections with Congo red. In addition to the obvious eosinophilic deposits identified by hematoxylin and eosin, Congo red staining of this lung tissue showed that additional amyloid was deposited in almost all sections of the alveolar wall. Given this patient's marked amyloidosis of both the lungs and the heart, it is not surprising that she experienced severe shortness of breath.

CASE

with a chief complaint of increasing shortness of breath. Blood gas studies revealed CO_2 retention, and she was intubated. Laboratory studies showed a slight elevation of serum calcium and a decrease of serum albumin. On the second day of hospitalization, the patient suffered cardiac arrest and died one hour later, approximately ten months after her initial presentation.[10]

Autopsy confirmed diffuse plasmacytosis of the bone marrow, consistent with multiple myeloma and showing many immature plasma cells. Every organ examined had amyloid deposits in the media of both arteries and veins. In several organs, including the heart, gastrointestinal tract, and diaphragm, amyloid deposits were also noted to be filling the vascular spaces and thus occluding the vessels (Figs. 9-2 and 9-3). Large focal deposits were also found in the wall of the left ventricle and in the intestinal mucosa. Postmortem studies of the kidney showed glomerular deposits of amyloid and Bence-Jones casts in the tubules. A striking feature of this case was diffuse amyloidosis in the alveolar septi of the lungs (Fig. 9-4). The cause of death was multiple myeloma and secondary amyloidosis. Amyloid involvement of myocardial fibers and vessels led to infarction and heart failure. Diffuse pulmonary amyloidosis explains the pulmonary hypertension and predominant right-sided heart failure.[11]

DISCUSSION

preted. The confirmed presence of amyloid in finger, gingival, and rectal tissue suggested that the amyloidosis was widespread. Amyloidosis of the heart and lungs probably caused the cardiac and pulmonary findings. Amyloid deposition in the kidneys may damage glomeruli and exacerbate the loss of serum proteins, including both albumin and the free lambda light chains, to the urine. Multiple myeloma often causes lytic lesions in bone. Such lytic lesions were not explicitly noted in this patient's clinical record, but may still have been present. If lytic lesions were present, they may have contributed to the patient's hypercalcemia.

10. The patient's fragile cardiac status was indicated by the fact that her failure to take her diuretic apparently led to her death. Her acute respiratory insufficiency may have been due to a variety of causes, including cardiac amyloidosis leading to cardiac failure with or without significant pulmonary edema, amyloidosis of the lungs, or a new process such as pneumonia or pulmonary embolism superimposed on her existing pulmonary disease. A cardiac arrest in a patient such as this one may be related to either the primary cardiac disease or an impairment of cardiac function secondary to severe hypoxia.

11. Amyloid is often found perivascularly and in the media of medium- to large-sized vessels. When the deposition significantly involves the vessel lumen, organ damage can occur. The deposition of amyloid in the cardiac parenchyma can cause restrictive cardiomyopathy and may have caused the hypoplastic left ventricle observed clinically. The less involved right ventricle was still sufficiently distensible to become somewhat enlarged and dilated. Large deposits of amyloid in the gastrointestinal mucosa did not produce prominent gastrointestinal symptoms. In contrast to other organs, even modest amyloid deposition in the glomerular capillary bed can produce significant clinical disease. Bence-Jones casts are precipitated immunoglobulin light chains within the renal tubules. The usual pattern of amyloid involvement of the lungs, when it occurs, is an involvement of medium-sized vessels. Extensive involvement of both the capillary bed and the alveolar walls is an unusual feature of this case that may have contributed to this patient's rapid decline.

Multiple Myeloma

Multiple myeloma is an uncontrolled proliferation of plasma cells. It is characterized by production of an immunoglobulin, often IgG or IgA, but occasionally also IgD or IgE. The onset of myeloma is often insidious, and patients may have only nonspecific complaints suggestive of chronic disease, such as weakness, anorexia, and weight loss. Excessive numbers of plasma cells in the blood are usually not present since the plasma cells tend to be confined to bone marrow and other organs including the spleen, liver, and lymph nodes. Erythrocyte, leukocyte, and platelet counts may be reduced if extensive plasmacytosis has occurred in the marrow. Such low counts may produce the expected complications of anemia, susceptibility to infection, and bleeding diatheses. Extensive plasmacytosis in marrow may also cause painful lytic bone lesions visible on radiographs. Light-chain immunoglobulin precursors, if made in excess, are sometimes found in the urine as Bence-Jones proteins. Damage to the kidney by the deposition of immunoglobulin can lead to renal failure with consequent elevated levels of blood urea nitrogen and creatinine. Multiple myeloma is still an almost uniformly fatal cancer, although radiation and chemotherapy can extend the typical patient's life span from less than two years to four or more years.

In a relatively small percentage of patients with multiple myeloma, light chains or their fragments are deposited in the tissues as a web of fibrils that are visible by electron microscopy and are known as amyloid. Patients with multiple myeloma who have amyloidosis tend to have a more aggressive clinical course than patients without amyloidosis. Deposition of amyloid in blood vessels can cause ischemia or infarction in tissues supplied by the blood vessels. Deposition of amyloid in the parenchyma of various organs may cause damage from pressure effects. The heart and kidneys are particularly vulnerable to amyloid deposition, and cardiac or renal insufficiency often dominates the clinical picture. Amyloid deposition in glomeruli may lead to breaks in the glomerular filtration system accompanied by protein loss to the urine and subsequent nephrotic syndrome. In addition to the amyloidosis associated with multiple myeloma, deposition of amyloid can occur idiopathically, in familial forms, or secondary to chronic inflammatory conditions.

Questions

1. What is multiple myeloma? How does it produce symptoms? What symptoms can it produce? What is amyloidosis? What is the relationship between multiple myeloma and amyloidosis? How does amyloidosis produce symptoms?
2. How did this patient present? Describe the variety of complaints she experienced. At what point is it appropriate to conclude that a single underlying disease might account for most or all of her problems?
3. How were multiple myeloma and amyloidosis diagnosed in this patient? How are these diagnoses related to the problems the patient experienced? How did she die? What was found at autopsy?

Selected Reading

Barlogie B, Epstein J, Selvanayagam P, Alexanian R: Plasma cell myeloma — new biological insights and advances in therapy. Blood 73:865–879, 1989.

Hawkins PN: Amyloidosis. Blood Rev 2:270–280, 1988.

10 AIDS IN A PATIENT WITH HEMOPHILIA

Key Words | hemophilia, AIDS, immunocompromised host

CASE

A 53-year-old male patient with hemophilia was admitted from the emergency room because of increasing shortness of breath. The shortness of breath, together with exacerbation of a chronic cough and occasional blood-stained sputum, had been developing during the six weeks preceding admission. The major manifestation of the patient's hemophilia throughout his life had been the occurrence of hemarthroses every few weeks. The patient had feared the possibility of contracting acquired immune deficiency syndrome (AIDS) and had therefore tried for several years to limit his use of factor VIII concentrates.[1] Bone marrow studies had been performed two years previously because of anemia and pancytopenia during a bout of hepatitis B. These studies demonstrated findings that were considered at that time to be consistent with a preleukemic syndrome. Subsequent testing, however, had revealed a normal leukocyte karyotype.[2]

Vital signs early in the final admission included a temperature of 38.3°C (normal, 37.0°C), respiratory rate of 26/min (normal resting rate, 6 to 20/min), heart rate of 110/min (normal resting rate, 60 to 100/min) and regular, and a blood pressure within normal limits. Rales were detected in the chest and lungs, without dullness, bilaterally from the base to approximately one-third of the lung fields. Arterial blood gases on room air included a pH of 7.5 (normal, pH 7.38 to 7.44), PCO_2 25 mmHg (normal, 35 to 45 mmHg), and PO_2 30 mmHg (normal, 80 to 100 mmHg).[3] On 40% face mask oxygen, the arterial blood gases were pH

DISCUSSION

1. Increasing shortness of breath accompanied by cough and blood-stained sputum suggests processes such as pneumonia, tumor, or pulmonary congestion. The bleeding in hemophilia occurs primarily into weight-bearing joints and muscles. This predilection may reflect commonly occurring minor trauma to these structures. Factor VIII concentrates, which are prepared from the serum of hundreds to thousands of donors, can reduce the danger of bleeding. Unfortunately, some patients who received these concentrates in the early 1980s, before procedures were initiated to screen for contaminated blood, were exposed to human immunodeficiency virus (HIV).

2. Hepatitis virus can also be present in blood products. It is consequently common for hemophiliac patients to have a history of hepatitis. Pancytopenia in a patient with hemophilia may increase the severity of the patient's bleeding diathesis if thrombocytopenia occurs. Many chronic leukemias develop slowly, and the boundary between the absence and presence of leukemia may be poorly defined. Abnormal chromosomes are often present in leukemic cell lines. The absence of an abnormal karyotype in this patient raises the possibility that the bone marrow signs were due to something other than a preleukemic syndrome.

3. Pneumonia was suggested by the patient's fever, increased respiration and heart rate, rales, and arterial blood gases. The arterial blood gases indicated that this patient was in a serious condition: the PO_2 was very low, and he was seriously alkalotic. The alkalosis was the result of hyperventilating and conse-

CASE

7.46, PCO_2 27 mmHg, and PO_2 48 mmHg. A chest radiograph demonstrated a right lower lobe consolidation. Bronchography demonstrated a diffuse alveolar process. A Gram-stained sputum sample contained gram-positive rods and cocci.[4]

Physical examination also revealed scleral icterus, palpable spleen, and a positive abdominal fluid wave. Liver function studies showed a total bilirubin of 5.3 mg/100 ml (normal, 0.3 to 1.5 mg/100 ml), a direct bilirubin of 4.3 mg/100 ml (normal, 0.1 to 0.4 mg/100 ml), normal total protein, and a serum albumin level of 2.3 g/100 ml (normal, 3.5 to 5.5 g/100 ml). The clinical impression was chronic pneumonia, possibly caused by *Legionella* or *Pneumocystis*.[5]

The patient was given intravenous antibiotics, and his condition appeared to improve over the next few days. The ratio of the patient's T-helper cells to T-suppressor cells was about 0.7 (normal, 1.15 to 3.20). This information, together with the patient's history of hemophilia, raised the possibility that he had AIDS.[6] His physical condition and respiratory status began to deteriorate four or five days after admission. Bronchial brushings demonstrated *Pneumocystis carinii*, and pentamidine, obtained from the Centers for Disease Control, was added to the therapy.[7]

One week after admission, the patient became unconscious. It was thought that the loss of consciousness might be due to a toxic metabolic state, probably secondary to intravenous morphine therapy that had been given to facilitate ventilator therapy. Narcan therapy did not, however, reverse the coma. Other diagnostic possibilities then included central nervous system infections with opportunistic organisms and a toxic metabolic state due to poor liver function. Computed tomography and lumbar puncture studies did not yield conclusive evidence of hemorrhage or infection. There was a suggestion of a left lateral temporal lobe lesion that might have represented a viral focus of infection, perhaps due to hepatitis B virus.[8]

The patient became severely hypotensive and died ten days after admission. Autopsy studies revealed *Pneumocystis* pneumonia and disseminated candidiasis (Fig. 10-1). *Candida* was found in the

DISCUSSION

quently lowering blood CO_2 levels with resulting loss of buffering capacity.

4. The patient's condition improved when he was given oxygen by face mask, but not as much as might have been hoped. The specific cause of pneumonia was still unclear several days after admission, since the radiograph and bronchogram findings were nonspecific and the Gram stain gave confusing results. Bronchograms are radiographic images made after a thin layer of contrast medium is inserted into the bronchi, usually via bronchoscopy. A thin, even coating of the inner surface of the bronchial tree can be obtained by systematically changing the patient's position.

5. Signs of hepatic dysfunction included low serum albumin, ascites, high levels of conjugated bilirubin, scleral icterus, and jaundice. These signs might have been due either to reactivation of hepatitis or simply to the increased metabolic demands of a serious infection. Both *Legionella* and *Pneumocystis* infections produce a severe pneumonia that can diffusely involve alveoli and may produce intra-alveolar hemorrhage. *Pneumocystis* is a protozoan that rarely infects previously healthy patients, but is common in patients with AIDS.

6. T-helper cells are selectively attacked by HIV, leading to a reversal of the normal T-helper cell to T-suppressor cell ratio. This case was an early AIDS case that occurred before the development of techniques for measuring serum antibodies to HIV. Infections in AIDS patients are notoriously difficult to treat because the immune system is compromised. The infections may be caused by bacterial, fungal, protozoal, or viral parasites. Reactivation of chronic viral infections, such as this patient's hepatitis B, is common. The patient's "preleukemic syndrome" two years previously can be reinterpreted as an early manifestation of AIDS.

7. The Centers for Disease Control in Atlanta, Georgia, are an important source in the United States for rarely used drugs and for experimental drugs that are not licensed for routine use. Usually, patients treated with experimental drugs must be enrolled in a therapeutic study. Pentamidine is an antibiotic with activity against *Pneumocystis carinii*; trimethoprim-sulfamethoxazole is an alternative therapy.

8. Unfortunately, it is fairly common for a serious sign,

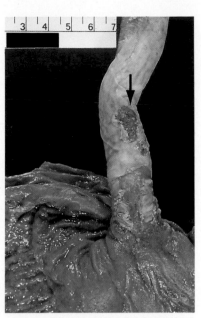

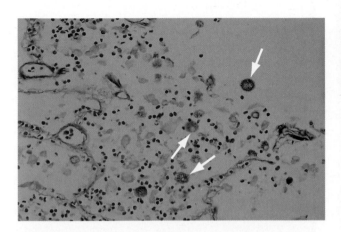

Fig. 10-1. *Pneumocystis* pneumonia (high power photomicrograph, Gomori methenamine silver [GMS]). The alveoli are filled with erythrocytes and leukocytes. Some leukocytes stain gray with GMS stain *(arrows)* because they contain clusters of *Pneumocystis* organisms.

Fig. 10-2. Esophageal erosion (gross photograph). The stomach and esophagus have been everted to show the mucosal surface. The esophageal mucosa has a prominent longitudinal lesion *(arrow);* this lesion contained the fungus *Candida* on microscopic examination.

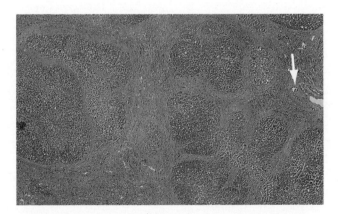

Fig. 10-3. Macronodular cirrhosis (low power photomicrograph, hematoxylin and eosin). The hepatic architecture shows various-sized nodules of functioning hepatocytes separated by broad fibrous bands. Since the biliary drainage is often disrupted by the fibrous bands, the nodules in cirrhotic livers are frequently green or yellow when observed grossly, and small collections of bile can be observed in microscopic sections under high power magnification. A remaining portal triad *(arrow)* is visible at the far right.

CASE

kidneys, hilar lymph nodes, esophagus, heart, and lungs (Fig. 10-2). No evidence of disseminated viral infection was found. The lymph nodes showed depleted T-cell zones. Extramedullary hematopoiesis was observed in the spleen and lymph nodes.[9]

On autopsy the liver was noted to be small (1,500 g) and showed macronodular cirrhosis (Fig. 10-3). Immunoperoxidase studies of microscopic sections from the liver were negative for hepatitis B core and surface antigens. Neuropathology studies showed bilirubin staining of the dura. No anatomical evidence of disease was found in the left lateral temporal lobe. A small infarction was found in the right cerebellum. Several microabcesses were found in the cerebral hemisphere, but no fungi or bacteria were identified.[10]

DISCUSSION

such as coma in this patient, to have several possible explanations, each of which has a different therapeutic implication.

9. An unsuspected opportunistic infection with the fungus *Candida* probably contributed to the patient's coma. It is also noteworthy that, contrary to clinical expectation, the patient did not have a reactivated hepatitis B infection secondary to AIDS. The depleted T-cell zones were one of the few anatomical findings directly reflecting the AIDS infection. Extramedullary hematopoiesis refers to the reproduction and maturation of blood cells outside the bone marrow. It is a relatively nonspecific finding, which occurs in people in whom marrow synthesis is inadequate.

10. The hepatic findings are consistent with the history of hepatitis B infection. The absence of evidence of hepatitis B surface or core antigen indicates that the patient's hepatitis B infection was not active and may no longer have been present. Bile staining of the dura is common in patients with jaundice. Hepatic encephalopathy may either cause or contribute to coma. The presence of cerebral microabcesses, in which no organism was identifiable, suggests that cerebral infection may have occurred but responded to antibiotic therapy. The patient's small cerebellar infarction might have been clinically insignificant even if he had not been comatose.

AIDS

HIV, the virus responsible for AIDS, is an RNA virus that infects human lymphocytes. It is able to infect a variety of cells in vitro, but has a marked predilection in vivo for lymphocytes known as T-helper cells. In these cells, virus infection can lead to marked cell abnormality, which is followed by the death of most, but probably not all, cells. The cells not killed by the infection probably act as reservoir for the disease. T-helper cells normally make up approximately 65% of the peripheral blood T cells. T-suppressor cells make up most of the remainder. During infection with HIV, the numbers of T-helper cells are reduced to less than the numbers of

T-suppressor cells. This phenomenon is called *helper/suppressor ratio reversal* and is characteristic of AIDS infection.

HIV is transmitted via infected blood, semen, and possibly saliva. Clinical symptoms usually develop several years after exposure to the virus. Some patients do not develop symptoms, but can still transmit the virus to other people. Others develop an AIDS-related complex, which is characterized by nonspecific symptoms including swollen lymph glands, fever, night sweats, malaise, diarrhea, and loss of weight. The remaining patients develop the complete AIDS syndrome.

The most prominent feature of the complete AIDS syndrome is a marked susceptibility to infection. The infecting organisms are typically unusual organisms, which rarely produce serious infection in hosts who are not immunocompromised. This susceptibility is a direct result of the destruction of T-helper cells, since these cells are the effector cells for delayed hypersensitivity and also "help" B cells develop into plasma cells. Organisms encountered in AIDS patients include protozoa (*Pneumocystis carinii, Toxoplasma gondii, Isospora belli, Cryptosporidium*), fungi (*Candida albicans, Cryptococcus neoformans, Coccidioides immitis, Histoplasma capsulatum*), bacteria (*Mycobacterium avium, Mycobacterium tuberculosis, Listeria monocytogenes, Nocardia asteroides, Salmonella*), and viruses (cytomegalovirus, herpes simplex virus, adenovirus, hepatitis B virus). AIDS patients also have a markedly increased susceptibility to certain cancers: 40% of homosexual AIDS patients develop either the vascular tumor called Kaposi's sarcoma (90%) or malignant lymphomas (10%).

Questions

1. By what method did this patient acquire AIDS? In what ways can clinical AIDS present? What is the significance of the patient's helper/suppressor ratio? What was found during his hepatitis B infection that was later reinterpreted to be an early manifestation of AIDS?

2. What evidence for infection did this patient have at his final admission? Which features suggested serious pulmonary disease? Which other organ systems were involved?

3. Which organisms were suspected as causing this patient's infection? To which other organisms are AIDS patients particularly vulnerable? How was infection proved and then treated? Discuss the patient's hospital course. What complications developed? What was found at autopsy?

Selected Reading

Masur H: Problems in the management of opportunistic infections in patients infected with human immunodeficiency virus. J Infect Dis 161:858–864, 1990.

Ragni MV, Nimorwicz P: Human immunodeficiency virus transmission and hemophilia. Arch Intern Med 149:1379–1380, 1989.

Redfield RR, Burke DS: HIV infection: the clinical picture. Sci Am 259(4):90–98, 1988.

Scutchfield FD, Benson AS: AIDS update. Postgrad Med 85:289–294, 301–304, 1989.

11 ACUTE LYMPHOCYTIC LEUKEMIA

Key Words | *leukemia, sarcoidosis, immunocompromised host*

CASE

Sarcoidosis was diagnosed in a 25-year-old black woman after biopsy of lymph nodes affected by mediastinal adenopathy.[1] Acute lymphocytic leukemia was diagnosed 14 months later (Fig. 11-2).[2] The patient was then treated with a wide variety of chemotherapeutic agents. The first treatment was leukapheresis followed by combined therapy with prednisone, vincristine, and cytosine arabinoside.[3] Her condition was complicated by vincristine neurotoxicity. The vincristine was then replaced by daunomycin. One month later, she was treated with a seven-day course of cytosine arabinoside and developed pancytopenia. Three months after diagnosis, therapy with cyclophosphamide, doxorubicin, methotrexate, and prednisone was started.[4] The patient presented two weeks later with a five-day history of low-grade fever, diarrhea, and hemoptysis. She was also noted to have a decline in her mental status.[5]

The patient was noted during physical examination to be cachectic and in moderate respiratory distress. Vital signs included blood pressure of 80/5 mmHg (normal, 100 to 140/60 to 90 mmHg), heart rate of 120/min (normal, 60 to 100/min), respiratory rate of 24/min (normal, 6 to 20/min), and temperature of 37.7°C (normal 37.0°C). The patient had lost much of her hair. The temporal muscles were wasted. She had an orocutaneous lesion consistent with oral candidiasis.[6] Breath sounds were diminished at the left base. Bilateral rales and rhonchi, most severe on the left, were present. The patient knew who she was but did

DISCUSSION

1. Sarcoidosis is a chronic granulomatous disease of unknown cause, somewhat similar to tuberculosis in histological appearance, that characteristically affects the lungs and mediastinal nodes. It is more common in black patients.

2. The relationship between the diagnosis of sarcoidosis in this patient and the diagnosis of acute leukemia less than 18 months later may be coincidental or may be due to an unrecognized interaction between the diseases. It is important to be aware of associations of this type, even though they are initially often vague and poorly documented, because they sometimes provide clues to the nature of the underlying processes of one or both diseases. In this case, sarcoidosis is known to be associated with abnormal T-lymphocyte numbers and functions, so there may be a relationship with the patient's later lymphocytic leukemia.

3. In the first step of leukapheresis therapy, blood is removed from the patient. The leukocytes are next separated from the remainder of the blood, often by centrifuging the blood. In the final step, the leukocyte-depleted blood is transfused back into the patient.

4. The patient's multiple drug regimens illustrate an important, limiting problem in the chemotherapy of many tumors. Cancer cells are similar to normal cells, and agents that kill cancer cells are often highly toxic to other cells. The degree of this toxicity varies from patient to patient, and chemotherapy often involves increasing the doses of several drugs until toxic levels are produced. The most toxic component of the regimen is then identified (usually by noting which side effect was most severe); if the dose of that agent is still

CASE

not know her location or the date. She was emotionally labile. The neurological examination was otherwise unremarkable. A chest radiograph revealed a right hilar density and a left lower lobe air/fluid level consistent with a pulmonary abscess or loculated pleural fluid. Cerebrospinal fluid was normal. Laboratory studies showed a hematocrit of 21% (normal, 35 to 47%), a white blood cell count of 900/mm³ (normal, 4,500 to 11,000/mm³), and a platelet count of 43,000/mm³ (normal, 150,000 to 450,000/mm³). Results of other laboratory studies were within normal limits.[7]

The patient was admitted and was treated with the antibiotics clindamycin and pipercillin. She received many blood transfusions.[8] She continued to be delirious and to experience visual hallucinations. Results of a bone marrow biopsy one week after admission were consistent with remission. Three days later, the patient underwent plasmapheresis, which resulted in an increase in the platelet count. Plasmapheresis was continued over the next several days.[9] Computed tomography performed the same day as the bone marrow biopsy revealed a probable abscess in the left par-

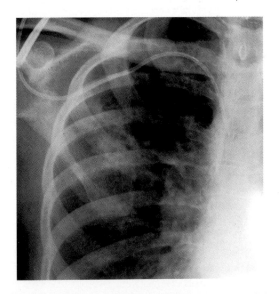

Fig. 11-1. Chest radiograph shows round, peripheral infiltrates seen most prominently in the patient's right upper lobe. Such infiltrates can be seen in pulmonary aspergillosis.

DISCUSSION

too low to be effective, the therapeutic regimen is modified by replacing the drug. Unfortunately, it is usually not possible to predict which toxic effects will be limiting in a particular patient.

5. Patients with leukemia are very vulnerable to infection because the leukemic cells are not able to perform their normal roles. The leukemic cells also occupy the bulk of the bone marrow at the expense of other cell lines. The patient's fever, diarrhea, and hemoptysis suggest that she had an infection. Her declining mental status was a sign of serious concern.

6. Low diastolic blood pressure, tachypnea, and tachycardia suggested that the patient was experiencing sepsis. Hair loss was probably the result of chemotherapy. Wasted temporal muscles reflect longstanding poor health. The possible presence of oral candidiasis warned that this patient was very vulnerable to opportunistic infections.

7. The chest examination and chest radiograph suggest that infection of the lung was present. This patient's neurological findings consisted of declining mental function without focal neurological changes or alterations in cerebrospinal fluid. Diagnostic possibilities included leukemic involvement of the brain and neurotoxicity due to one or more of the chemotherapeutic agents. The finding of normal cerebrospinal fluid tends to exclude bacterial infection of the meninges. However, since the patient was immunocompromised by both the leukemia and its therapy, nervous system infection by fungi or viruses, and bacterial infection of the brain parenchyma, were also diagnostic possibilities. The finding of pancytopenia suggests that chemotherapy caused suppression of normal bone marrow precursors as well as controlling the leukemia.

8. Clindamycin is effective against anaerobic bacteria. Pipericillin is a synthetic penicillin that has a broad spectrum of activity. The two drugs together were intended to be active against any pneumonia or abscess that the patient might have had. Unfortunately, neither drug is active against fungi. The repeated transfusions were designed to try to restore blood cells and platelets.

9. Plasmapheresis involves removing blood, centrifuging it to separate the plasma, discarding the plasma, resuspending the cells in an appropriate fluid or

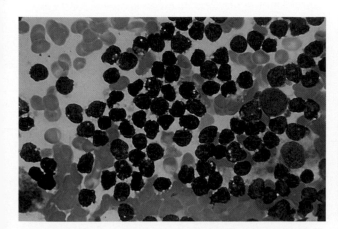

Fig. 11-2. Acute lymphocytic leukemia (high power photomicrograph, Wright's stain, from another case). This peripheral smear shows large numbers of lymphocytes (dark, round nuclei) and erythrocytes (lighter cells). Only a few other cells are visible.

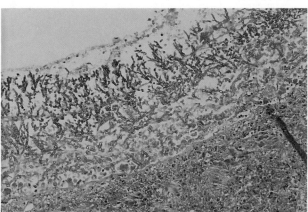

Fig. 11-3. *Aspergillus* invading bronchus (high power photomicrograph, hematoxylin and eosin). The wall of this bronchus has been almost completely destroyed by masses of the branching fungus. The surrounding alveoli were filled with hemorrhage and necrotic debris.

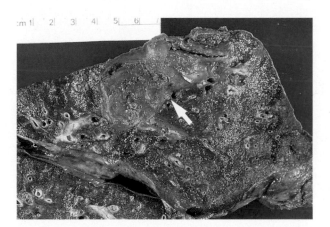

Fig. 11-4. Pulmonary sarcoidosis (gross photograph). A dense lesion *(arrow)* is visible grossly; it contained granulomatous tissue, consistent with sarcoidosis, when histological sections were examined.

CASE

ietomedial brain. Throat and stool cultures were positive for *Candida*. A chest radiograph taken three weeks after admission demonstrated left pneumothorax. Round, peripheral infiltrates present bilaterally were consistent with aspergillosis (Fig. 11-1). Percutaneous biopsy of the left lower lobe abscess five days later revealed *Aspergillus*. Amphotericin B therapy was started. Over the next few days, the patient's respiratory status progressively declined and she required increasing oxygen concentrations to maintain oxygenation. She was found dead approximately one month after admission.[10]

The autopsy examination was limited to the left lung.[11] An abscess (8 × 6 × 6 cm) was present in the left lower lobe. The entire lung weighed 600 g, and numerous firm hemorrhagic nodules were scattered throughout the parenchyma. Microscopic examination revealed extensive *Aspergillus* pneumonia and necrotizing obstructing bronchitis in all lobes (cultures were positive for *Aspergillus fumigatus*) (Fig. 11-3). Granulomatous lesions consistent with sarcoidosis were also observed in the pulmonary parenchyma (Fig. 11-4). In summary, at autopsy this patient was a 27-year-old black woman who had acute lymphocytic leukemia and who was severely immunocompromised as a result of her disease and the effects of chemotherapy; she had developed *Aspergillus* pneumonia, which ultimately proved fatal.[12]

DISCUSSION

plasma, and then transfusing the cells back into the patient. It is sometimes helpful, as in this case, in removing antibodies, metabolites, drugs, or toxins that are poisoning platelets or megakaryocytes, and consequently it can improve platelet lifespan.

10. The patient had documented *Candida* in the throat and *Aspergillus* in the lungs. Amphotericin B has activity against these opportunistic fungi. The probable brain abscess suggests that dissemination of either *Candida* or *Aspergillus*, or perhaps some other unsuspected opportunistic infection, may have occurred. Unfortunately, by the time the amphotericin B therapy was started, the patient was already so ill that her life could not be saved.

11. Often, with a little intelligent concern by the physician who requests the autopsy, both the legitimate concerns of the family and the legitimate needs of medicine for a more complete examination can be met. Limitation of the autopsy to a specific incision, rather than to examination of only the left lung, might have permitted a more complete examination.

12. *Aspergillus* produces a characteristic infection in which the bulk of the fungus grows in the air spaces and produces a dense mass of fungus (the so-called *fungus ball*) that can occlude the airways. Although such masses are not prominent in this case, they are highly allergenic in some patients and are sometimes diagnosed by the presence of intractable allergies and asthma. The granuloma produced by sarcoidosis is typically noncaseating and may show multiple giant cells. In time, the granulomas become replaced with hyaline fibrous scars.

Acute Lymphocytic Leukemia

Physical findings in acute lymphocytic leukemia can include enlarged lymph nodes, splenomegaly, and hepatomegaly. Fatigue is the most common symptom. Bone pain can also occur as a result of infiltration of the marrow by leukemic cells. This replacement leads to diminished production of normal cells by the bone marrow. Anemia, producing pallor, weakness, and rare cardiopulmonary compromise, may result. There is often also a loss of neutrophils and normal lymphocytes; the resulting inadequate numbers predispose the patient to frequent infections that may cause fever, pain, and loss of function of affected tissues. Purpura and hemorrhage are associated with low platelet counts.

Although the patient's symptoms at the time of presentation with an acute leukemia are often nonspecific, a blood smear is often done as part of the patient's evaluation and is usually diagnostic. Contrary to popular impression, the white blood cell count in patients with acute leukemia is not always markedly elevated, but instead can vary markedly. Somewhat fewer than one-third of patients have white blood cell counts of greater than $50,000/mm^3$, and about one-fifth have counts of less than $5000/mm^3$. In all patients, the majority of cells are usually recognizable leukemic cells. Bone marrow biopsy confirms the diagnosis. Chemotherapy of acute leukemias can be very effective; it has permitted prolonged remissions in adults with acute myelogenous leukemia and apparently true cures in many children with acute lymphocytic leukemia. The adult form of acute lymphocytic leukemia is often more refractory to therapy and tends also to be a disease of T lymphocytes rather than the more common B lymphocytes.

Questions

1. What type of leukemia did this patient have? How was it treated? What chemotherapeutic complications did she experience? What does her experience tell you about the toxicity of chemotherapeutic agents?

2. Why did this patient present to the hospital? What problems did her physical examination identify? Which organ systems were affected?

3. How did this patient's neurological status change with time? What factors contributed to her changing status? How did her respiratory status change with time? What respiratory problems did she develop? What was found at autopsy?

Selected Reading

Hayoe FG: Classification of acute leukaemias. Blood Rev 2:186–193, 1988.

Johns CJ, Scott PP, Schonfeld SA: Sarcoidosis. Annu Rev Med 40:353–371, 1989.

Kimmelman CP: Fungal infections in the immunocompromised patient. Ear Nose Throat J 67:852–855, 1988.

12 PULMONARY ASPERGILLOSIS IN A PATIENT WITH CHRONIC MYELOGENOUS LEUKEMIA

Key Words | *leukemia, aspergillosis, respiratory failure*

CASE

The patient was a 65-year-old man with Philadelphia chromosome-positive chronic myelogenous leukemia diagnosed six months previously (Fig. 12-1). At presentation, he had a leukocyte count of 54,000/mm³ (normal, 4,500 to 11,000/mm³) that consisted predominantly of neutrophils with approximately 5% immature blast forms (normal, 0 to 5%).[1] Since that time, the patient had lost weight. He had also noticed that he bruised easily, had occasional nosebleeds, and tended to bleed from hemorrhoids. The present admission was for chemotherapy.[2]

Physical examination revealed an apparently healthy man in no acute distress. No adenopathy was noted. Chest and neurological findings were within normal limits. Abdominal examination revealed mild hepatomegaly without splenomegaly. Admission laboratory data revealed a leukocyte count of 76,000/mm³ with a predominance of lymphocytes (61%; normal, 20 to 40%) as well as promyelocytes and blast forms (32%; normal, 0 to 5%).[3] The hematocrit was 22% (normal, 40 to

DISCUSSION

1. Patients with chronic myelogenous leukemia are typically middle-aged or older adults. The Philadelphia chromosome is a marker for the disease. Chronic myelogenous leukemia tends to present as a chronic disease, which may later develop into an acute leukemia. In the chronic phase, mature granulocytes (mostly neutrophils) usually predominate in the peripheral smear. Only a small percentage of the cells are immature forms.

2. A decrease in weight is common in patients with cancer. The reasons for this are unknown. A coagulopathy, possibly due to decreased platelet synthesis by leukemic marrow, is suggested by easy bruising, nosebleeds, and bleeding from hemorrhoids.

3. Most patients with chronic myelogenous leukemia do not show adenopathy. Massive splenomegaly occurs in some patients, but may be reduced with chemotherapy. Blast crisis occurs when an indolent, chronic leukemia changes to a more acute form. Blast crises are characterized by a shift in the predominant leukemic cells from mature to less mature ("blast") forms.

73

CASE

52%). The platelet count was 13,000/mm^3 (normal, 150,000 to 450,000/mm^3). Prothrombin and partial thromboplastin times were within normal limits. A chest radiograph showed normal heart and lungs. The impression at admission was chronic myelogenous leukemia with blast crisis.[4]

The patient's chronic myelogenous leukemia was treated with high-dose cytosine arabinoside to induce remission. All cell counts decreased as expected; he was transfused with multiple blood products, and empirical antibiotic therapy was started. As a result of pancytopenia, the patient developed hemorrhoidal bleeding, oral candidiasis, and bilateral lung infiltrates.[5] Three weeks after chemotherapy, his bone marrow had not recovered. Amphotericin B was added to the medications because of a sustained low-grade fever. Cultures of stool, sputum, and urine grew *Candida*. A culture of specimens from the oral cavity grew herpes simplex virus. Intravenous acyclovir therapy was begun.[6]

One month after admission, the patient's marrow was beginning to show recovery, but there was no improvement in his respiratory status. *Aspergillus* was found in sputum and bronchoalveolar lavage cultures.[7] Concurrently, the patient developed a right maxillary sinus fluid level. He became hypotensive and experienced bronchospasm following treatment with amphotericin B. He was transferred to an intensive care unit because of increased respiratory difficulties. At approximately the same time, his mental status deteriorated significantly. The results of a lumbar puncture were unremarkable, and a cerebrospinal fluid culture was sterile. A computed tomogram of the head was also normal, but a repeated scan revealed multiple white matter lucencies in both hemispheres. The patient's condition continued to deteriorate, and he died.[8]

At autopsy, the patient's bone marrow was noted to be hypocellular and consisted predominantly of myeloid forms (Fig. 12-2). In the spleen, only scant white pulp was seen. There was also severe sinusoidal congestion and scattered hemosiderin throughout the spleen.[9] Several infarcted

DISCUSSION

4. The shift toward immature forms can be accompanied by a pancytopenia of other marrow lines since the marrow is overwhelmed by the leukemic cell line. In many patients, the acute leukemia is from the B lymphocyte cell line rather than the granulocyte cell line.

5. Cytosine arabinoside, also known as ara C or cytarabine, is a pyrimidine analog that is useful in the control of blast crisis. Cytosine arabinoside causes substantial bone marrow suppression of normal cell lines as well. The balance between dangerous marrow suppression and control of the leukemia is delicate. Patients are vulnerable to infection for various periods after chemotherapy. Transfusions are used to maintain red blood cell and platelet counts. Antibiotics protect the patient from bacterial infection. Unfortunately, many organisms, particularly fungi and viruses but also antibiotic-resistant bacteria, are not susceptible to broad-spectrum antibiotics.

6. Failure of the bone marrow to begin recovery within a few weeks may be a dangerous prognostic sign since it indicates that bone marrow suppression of normal constituents is excessive. The bone marrow sometimes, but not always, will recover later. When this patient developed a fever, the toxic antifungal agent amphotericin B was promptly added to the regimen because fungal infection was feared. Culture results later confirmed that the patient had developed both widespread fungal (*Candida*) and herpesvirus infections. Amphotericin B is effective against *Candida*. Acyclovir has some activity, but not as much as might be desired, against herpesvirus. Most probably, the patient harbored the *Candida* as part of his flora and had been previously exposed to herpesvirus and then retained it in latent form.

7. Evidence of a second fungal infection, due to *Aspergillus*, was found by bronchial washings one week later. Unfortunately the patient's *Aspergillus* infection appeared to be more resistant to antifungal therapy than was the *Candida* infection. *Aspergillus* is a ubiquitous fungus whose portal of entry is the respiratory tract. In a healthy host, the fungus tends to be confined to the airways and does not actually infect the tissues. True *Aspergillus* infection can occur in immunocompromised hosts. The major factor in

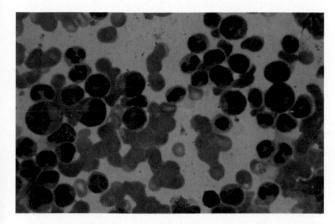

Fig. 12-1. Chronic myelogenous leukemia (high power photomicrograph, from another case, Wright's stain). This peripheral smear, taken during a blast crisis, shows large numbers of immature precursors of neutrophils.

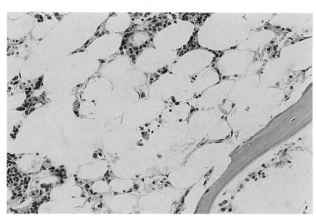

Fig. 12-2. Hypocellular bone marrow (high power photomicrograph, hematoxylin and eosin). Aggressive chemotherapy has markedly decreased the cellularity of this bone marrow specimen, taken at autopsy, in all cell lines. Such a decrease in marrow precursor cells can produce clinical pancytopenia.

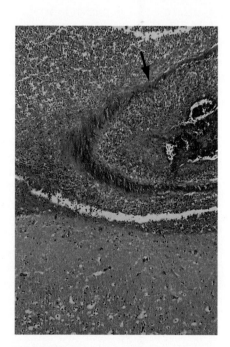

Fig. 12-3. *Aspergillus* invading vessel wall (low power photomicrograph, hematoxylin and eosin). The wall of a meningeal vessel has been heavily invaded by the fungus; the arrow marks the boundary between normal vessel wall *(above right)* and vessel infiltrated with *Aspergillus*. The vessel is occluded by clot and debris; substantial hemorrhage and debris is present in the meninges as well. Compare with Fig. 11-2 showing *Aspergillus* invading a bronchus.

CASE

areas of the lungs contained septated hyphae morphologically characteristic of *Aspergillus*. The fungi were found in vessels, on the pleural surface, and invading the chest wall. Microscopically, blood vessel invasion was extensively demonstrated in the lungs. Foci containing *Aspergillus* were also found in the heart and thyroid. Little inflammatory infiltrate accompanied areas of *Aspergillus* invasion in the lung, and only a mild reaction was seen to foci in the heart and thyroid.[10] The cerebral hemispheres contained multiple areas of hemorrhagic encephalomalacia. Microscopic examination of these areas revealed cortical necrosis and invasion of blood vessel walls by *Aspergillus* (Fig. 12-3). Some of the cerebral vessels were thrombosed. In contrast to the mild reactions seen in the heart and thyroid, neutrophils were abundant in the area of cortical necrosis. The ventricular system showed multiple petechial hemorrhage and contained a purulent exudate. The cause of death was considered to be respiratory failure in a patient with chronic myelogenous leukemia complicated by disseminated aspergillosis.[11]

DISCUSSION

host susceptibility to *Aspergillus* infection is granulocytopenia. Disseminated aspergillosis can invade vessel walls. This invasion can then cause thrombosis and infarction.

8. The right maxillary sinus fluid level was probably observed either by transillumination of the sinuses or by radiography of the head. Its presence suggests that a sinus infection is present. Amphotericin B is a toxic, complex drug whose administration is associated with a high incidence of allergic and other adverse reactions. Both poor respiratory status and cortical necrosis probably contributed to deteriorating mental status.

9. The hypocellular marrow is the histological correlate of the clinically observed pancytopenia. The predominance of myeloid forms suggests that the anemia and thrombocytopenia may have been more severe than the leukopenia. Scant splenic white pulp is secondary to lymphocyte destruction during chemotherapy. Chronic myelogeneous leukemia can produce massive splenomegaly, predominantly by impairing normal splenic circulation. After the destruction of the white pulp, the congested sinuses remain as evidence of the previous splenomegaly. The presence of hemosiderin suggests that intrasplenic hemorrhage may have occurred.

10. Blood vessel invasion by *Aspergillus* indicates that the fungus was spreading by a hematological route. Since *Aspergillus* is a highly antigenic organism, such spread is rare in patients who are not immunocompromised. The lack of inflammatory infiltrate around the foci of *Aspergillus* confirms that the patient's immunocompromised state was a factor in permitting the fungus to become established in his tissues.

11. Foci of *Aspergillus* in vessels can form a surface upon which thrombosis occurs. Resulting small areas of infarctions in the cortical white matter are observed as pale areas, known as *encephalomalacia*. The reason for the more vigorous immune response to the *Aspergillus* in the brain and ventricles is unclear, but is perhaps the result of selective survival of neutrophils in the brain parenchyma secondary to lower concentrations of cytosine arabinoside in cerebral spinal fluid than in plasma.

Chronic Myelogenous Leukemia

In chronic myelogenous leukemia, there is an increased production of all granulocyte lines, although neutrophils typically predominate. The disease has been strongly associated with a characteristic chromosome marker, known as the Philadelphia chromosome. This marker is detected by chromosome analysis of peripheral blood and bone marrow. The marker is a reciprocal translocation between the long arms of chromosomes 22 and 9. The link between the translocation and the disease appears to be that rearrangement creates a fusion gene product with enzymatic activity as a tyrosine kinase. Chronic myelogenous leukemia is one of the first tumors in which the relationship between chromosomal damage and pathophysiology is beginning to be understood in some detail.

Chronic myelogenous leukemia usually presents with splenomegaly, which may be marked, and an elevation in the white blood cell count. Splenomegaly occurs because of proliferation of granulocytes in the spleen. Later in the disease, extramedullary hematopoiesis can also occur in liver sinusoids to produce hepatomegaly. The patient may be asymptomatic; in this case the diagnosis is made as an incidental laboratory finding. Alternatively, the enlarged spleen may have produced left upper quadrant discomfort, which may lead a patient to consult a physician. Anemia, weight loss, fever, or arthralgias may also have prompted the patient to seek medical attention. The Philadelphia chromosome, if present, is an important diagnostic clue. Low leukocyte alkaline phosphatase levels are also an important diagnostic clue. The enzyme is a normal constituent of granulocytes. It is present at reduced levels in almost all patients who are not infected and have not been treated with steroids. Successful therapy of the disease may also result in near normal levels of leukocyte alkaline phosphatase. Serum vitamin B_{12} levels can be increased. This increase is presumably due to the presence of increased levels of transcobalamin I, a vitamin B_{12}-binding protein produced by granulocytes. Increased cell turnover may produce hyperuricemia both before and during treatment. Glycolipid-laden macrophages may be present in the spleen and bone marrow.

Chronic myelogenous leukemia typically occurs in two distinct phases. In the chronic phase, a markedly elevated white blood cell count, which may exceed 200,000/mm³, may be present. This leukocytosis is characteristically composed of mature granulocytes, with no more than 5% of the cells being myeloblast forms. In this phase, the disease has an indolent course and a patient may appear quite healthy. However, the malignant clone is vulnerable to further mutations. These mutations can modify the disease and produce accelerated production of basophils and mature but dysplastic neutrophils. The percentage of granulocyte precursors in marrow and blood also increases. These changes tend to be accompanied by increasing resistance to chemotherapy. Finally, in many patients, progressive proliferation of blasts and other early myeloid elements may result in their completely dominating the marrow. The disease then behaves like an acute leukemia, and the patient is said to have entered a "blast crisis." The acute leukemia is most commonly of the myeloblastic form. However, in nearly one third of patients, the leukemia appears to be of B-lymphocyte lineage. This observation has been cited as evidence that the original transformed cell must be so primitive as to be able to give rise to both myeloid and lymphocytic cell lines.

Questions

1. What is the natural history of chronic myelogenous leukemia? What symptoms did this patient experience? What were his initial white cell count and differential? Why was the patient admitted?
2. How were the results of the patient's blood studies after admission different from those of his earlier studies? What was the significance of these differences? How was he treated? Was the treatment successful in inducing remission?
3. What complications did the patient develop as a consequence of pancytopenia? How were these complications treated? How did he die? What was found at autopsy?

Selected Reading

Canellos GP: Treatment of chronic granulomatous leukemia in blastic crisis. Bone Marrow Transplant 4(suppl. 1):131–132, 1989.

Shepherd PC, Ganesan TS, Galton DA: Haematological classification of the chronic myeloid leukemias. Baillieres Clin Haematol 1:887–906, 1987.

RESPIRATORY SYSTEM

13 MASSIVE PULMONARY EMBOLISM COMPLICATING OCCULT LYMPHOMA

Key Words | lymphoma, pulmonary embolism, sudden death

CASE

The patient was a 71-year-old man who was in excellent health until approximately one month before admission, when he noted upper respiratory symptoms of nasal congestion and dry cough. A left-sided pleuritic chest pain was present. He was treated with oral antibiotics, but his symptoms persisted.[1] Fever, chills, and night sweats along with anorexia and a 30-lb weight loss also occurred during this period. The cough persisted as a dry, hacking cough without hemoptysis. The patient was hospitalized and given intravenous cephalosporins, again without resolution of symptoms. Temperature elevations to 40°C (normal, 37°C) continued.[2] Computed tomography of the chest revealed bilateral pleural effusions with irregular densities and cavitation of the right upper lobe and apex (Fig. 13-1). The patient had never smoked but had worked as a coal miner for 30 years and had been diagnosed with black lung disease. He was transferred to a university hospital for evaluation of his pulmonary disease.[3]

The patient's lungs had decreased breath sounds at the left base and rhonchi in the right upper lobe with egophony. Lymph nodes were unremarkable. Extremities showed bilateral stasis dermatitis with varicose veins.[4] The hematocrit

DISCUSSION

1. A common cold, although not serious in itself, may become complicated by pneumonia in an elderly or debilitated patient. Pleuritic pain is characteristically sharp and accentuated during breathing. It is often associated with underlying lung disease such as pneumonia, tuberculosis, pulmonary infarction, or neoplasm. Failure to respond to antibiotics may indicate the presence of resistant organisms or a low concentration of antibiotic at the site of infection. Alternatively, some other pathological process, which may or may not be coexisting with infection, may be dominating the clinical picture.
2. The severity of the patient's symptoms, and particularly the pronounced weight loss, suggests that a serious disease such as cancer, tuberculosis, or leukemia may be present.
3. Pleural effusions are accumulations of fluid between the pleura and chest wall. Irregular densities suggest focal processes such as metastatic tumor or granulomatous disease. Cavitation is associated with necrosis and can occur in a variety of diseases, including abscess and tuberculosis. The history of coal mining suggests the presence of a risk factor for both lung cancer and chronic obstructive pulmonary disease. The dry cough and recent weight loss are usually not consistent with chronic bronchitis.

81

CASE

was 33% (normal, 40 to 52%). The leukocyte count was 28,900/mm[3] (normal, 4,500 to 11,000/mm[3]) with 30% neutrophils (normal, 40 to 70%) and 65% lymphocytes (normal, 20 to 40%). The peripheral blood smear was considered unremarkable.[5] Arterial blood gases on room air showed pH 7.46 (normal, pH 7.38 to 7.44), PO_2 59 mmHg (normal, 80 to 100 mmHg), and PCO_2 33 mmHg (normal, 35 to 45 mmHg). The most likely diagnosis for this patient was considered to be tuberculosis with cavitation, but a sputum sample contained no acid-fast bacilli. The patient had mildly elevated liver function tests, with alanine aminotransferase (SGPT) of 92 IU/L (normal < 37 IU/L) and aspartate aminotransferase (SGOT) of 155 IU/L (normal < 34 IU/L).[6] The differential diagnosis at this point included tuberculosis, metastatic cancer, lung carcinoma, fungal infection, chronic lymphocytic leukemia, and bacterial abscess.

That evening the patient became febrile with a temperature of 38.5°C. He had several minutes of substernal chest pain, which was relieved with nitroglycerine. No electrocardiographic recording was obtained at that time.[7] Two days later, the patient suddenly collapsed after standing to go to the bathroom. He complained of acute onset of dyspnea with chest pain followed by syncope.[8] The blood pressure was 80 mmHg/palpable (normal, 100 to 140/60 to 90 mmHg), the pulse was 110/min (normal resting pulse, 60 to 100/min), and the respiratory rate was 36/min (normal resting rate, 6 to 20/min). Blood gases showed pH 7.32, PCO_2 26 mmHg, and PO_2 56 mmHg on room air. Dopamine therapy was started, but the patient's blood pressure remained refractory. He became unresponsive and went into ventricular fibrillation; cardiopulmonary resuscitation was unsuccessful.[9]

At autopsy, a saddle embolus was found that occluded the major pulmonary arteries (Fig. 13-2). The remainder of the lung parenchyma showed areas of multiple infarctions (Fig. 13-3). There was evidence of well-differentiated lymphocytic lymphoma in retroperitoneal and pulmonary hilar lymph nodes, with additional involvement of bone marrow and liver (Fig. 13-4). A review of the

DISCUSSION

4. Decreased breath sounds occur in a variety of settings including obesity, obstructive lung disease, pleural effusion, and pneumothorax. Rhonchi suggest the presence of mucus. *Egophony* is an alteration in the filtration of sound through the chest such that a spoken "ee" is heard through a stethoscope as "ay." It may indicate solidification of lung tissue, fluid in the lung, or fluid in the pleural space. Swollen lymph nodes might have suggested either infection or involvement of the nodes by a process such as tumor or granulomatous disease. Stasis dermatitis refers to the thin and atrophic skin produced by venous insufficiency.

5. The patient's leukocytosis was composed predominantly of lymphocytes and would consequently be unusual in an acute bacterial infection, although it might be consistent with viral infection, chronic tuberculosis, or lymphocytic leukemia. The significance of this patient's normocytic, normochromic anemia is unclear, but either the anemia of chronic disease or anemia related to destruction of bone marrow is possible.

6. The patient has a mild respiratory alkalosis, possibly consistent with mild hyperventilation to partially correct for low arterial oxygen tension. Mycobacteria can be rare in sputum in active tuberculosis, so the absence of acid-fast bacilli in his sputum sample does not necessarily rule out the disease. Mildly elevated liver function tests suggest the possibility of liver metastasis.

7. Nitroglycerine characteristically relieves angina, but may also occasionally appear to relieve other types of chest pain that spontaneously subside within a few minutes. If possible, electrocardiographic recordings should be obtained during a period of chest pain to confirm the presence of changes consistent with myocardial ischemia.

8. This patient's history shows that he is susceptible to large pulmonary embolus: the thrombus forms in deep leg veins of a sick patient during prolonged bed rest and dislodges or breaks when the patient uses his legs to stand; then an embolus becomes entrapped in the pulmonary circulation, causing dyspnea, chest pain, and syncope. However, this symptom pattern has other causes that may lead to sudden death, including massive myocardial infarction, sudden onset of ventricular fibrillation, and

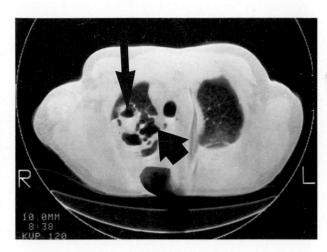

Fig. 13-1. Computed tomogram of the lung shows cavitation of the right apex *(arrows)* surrounded by areas of increased radiographic density. The cavitation in this patient was a consequence of pulmonary infarction, but can also be seen in tumors, tuberculosis, abscesses, and other pulmonary processes.

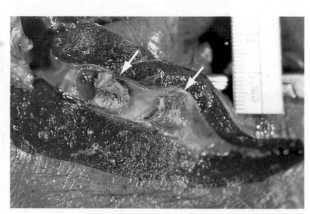

Fig. 13-2. Pulmonary embolus (lung, gross photograph from another case). A branch of the pulmonary artery has been opened to reveal two fragments of a pulmonary embolus *(arrows)* that were probably derived from a deep vein thrombus. The fragment on the left appears folded.

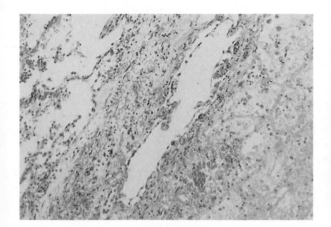

Fig. 13-3. Pulmonary infarction (low power photomicrograph, hematoxylin and eosin). The area of infarction is in the right of the field. In this region, the alveolar cells have died and their nuclei have disintegrated. The alveolar lumena are filled with lysed red blood cells and proteinaceous debris. In contrast, the healthy tissue in the left shows clear alveoli; the nuclei are preserved; and the capillaries are intact. The boundary between the infarcted and healthy lobules is marked by a diagonal band of fibrous tissue into which some hemorrhage has occurred.

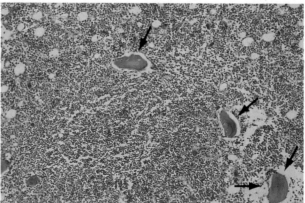

Fig. 13-4. Lymphoma involving bone marrow (low power photomicrograph, hematoxylin and eosin). A heavy, nodular, lymphocytic infiltration is present in the lower center of the field. Three small fragments of bone *(arrows)* are visible. The remaining marrow is hypercellular and has replaced many of the normal fat cells. Normal cell lines are present.

CASE

original peripheral blood smear showed the process to be present there as well. Anthracosilicosis was present, but was mild. The patient's pulmonary symptoms appear to have been due to pulmonary infarction rather than to infection or black lung disease. The right upper lobe contained an inflammatory cavitation process which appeared to be secondary to a previous pulmonary infarction. Neutrophils were the predominant inflammatory cells, with lymphocytes present in smaller numbers. No granulomas were seen. Hemorrhage and early fibrosis were seen around the periphery of the process. Prominent coronary atherosclerosis with cardiomegaly and biventricular hypertrophy was observed. The cause of death was considered to be massive pulmonary embolism complicating well-differentiated lymphocytic lymphoma.[10]

DISCUSSION

rupture of an aortic aneurysm. Many of these processes may be triggered by the sympathetic outflow or increased arterial pressure associated with the physiological correction of the hypotension produced by standing.

9. Rapid pulse and respiratory rate coupled with dropping blood pressure suggest impending cardiopulmonary arrest, possibly leading to death. The blood gases are consistent with metabolic acidosis partially compensated by hyperventilation. The presence of metabolic acidosis in this patient suggests that some process, possibly pulmonary infarction, has caused substantial tissue destruction. Resuscitation of a patient with massive pulmonary embolism may be impossible. Therapy with dopamine was given in case the patient's episode was of cardiac origin.

10. The phrase *saddle embolus* refers to a massive pulmonary embolus entrapped in the branch point of an artery in such a way that it occludes both branches. The presence of multiple infarctions suggests that the patient has had multiple previous pulmonary emboli. Repeated episodes of pulmonary embolism with infarction account for the history of fever, chills, cough, night sweats, and chest pain. Although lymphoma per se was not clinically suspected, the cells in well-differentiated lymphocytic lymphoma are very similar to those in chronic lymphocytic leukemia, and it is thought that the two diseases represent the same disease process occurring in different sites. The patient's lymphoma accounts for his weight loss and anorexia.

Pulmonary Emboli

Pulmonary emboli most commonly arise when a portion of a thrombus, typically from a deep vein in the leg, breaks off and is carried by the venous system through the right side of the heart to lodge in the pulmonary arterial system. Such thrombi form initially as a consequence of stasis in the venous system. Pulmonary emboli are probably very common, but most are small and cause no symptoms. In patients who do have symptomatic pulmonary embolic disease, several patterns emerge. Massive pulmonary emboli lodge early in the pulmonary arterial tree and can cause sudden death, as occurred in this patient. Intermediate-sized pulmonary emboli can cause pulmonary infarction by occluding the blood supply to a volume of lung large enough that collateral circulation is not adequate but small enough to avoid sudden death. Multiple small pulmonary emboli may produce increased pulmonary artery pressure as a result of the increased resistance to blood flow in the lungs. This increased pressure may cause right-sided heart failure. Some patients appear to have multiple episodes of small pulmonary emboli without developing either right-sided heart failure or infarction. These patients experience only repeated episodes of dyspnea and tachycardia accompanied by apprehension and chest pain.

Questions

1. What was the patient's clinical history before his transfer to a university hospital? What risk factors for pulmonary disease did he have? What symptoms did he experience? What were possible causes of his pulmonary symptoms? Which of his symptoms might have been due to disease in other organ systems?
2. What events happened during the patient's hospital course? What are possible explanations of these events? How was he treated? Were the treatments successful? Do you think that the patient received reasonable and appropriate care?
3. Discuss the findings that were consistent with the occult lymphocytic leukemia found at autopsy. What lessons about missed diagnoses do you learn from this case?

Selected Reading

Dunmire SM: Pulmonary embolism. Emerg Med Clin N Am 7:339–354, 1989.

Foon KA, Gale RP: Immunologic classification of lymphoma and lymphoid leukemia. Blood Rev 1:77–88, 1987

Mammen EF: Pathophysiology of thrombophilic states. Folia Haematol (Leipz) 115:243–252, 1988.

14 CHRONIC OBSTRUCTIVE PULMONARY DISEASE WITH COR PULMONALE

Key Words | COPD, cor pulmonale, seizures, mental status change

CASE

A 46-year-old man with a long history of chronic obstructive pulmonary disease, cor pulmonale, and pneumonia was admitted to a community hospital with pulmonary disease.[1] Intubation was required during the patient's 18-day hospital stay. Sputum cultures grew *Pseudomonas*, for which he was treated with antibiotics gentamicin and cefazolin. Two weeks after being discharged, the patient became suicidal. He attempted to shoot himself in the head and to slash his wrists with a screwdriver.[2] Several days later, he was brought to an emergency room in a stupor. His pupils were dilated and he had experienced what was considered to be an "ischemic seizure." He was tearful, confused, and affectively labile. He was sent home after he had apparently recovered. A similar episode occurred later in the day. He returned to the emergency room. He was transferred to a university hospital, where he had a third seizure and respiratory arrest. He was intubated and admitted to the hospital.[3]

The patient had a history of multiple admissions for pulmonary disease. He was admitted to a community hospital five times and to a university hospital twice during the year before his death. He had been unable to work during the preceding

DISCUSSION

1. The long history of pulmonary dysfunction suggests that this patient's respiratory status may be fragile. Pneumonia in patients with serious preexisting pulmonary disease is of great concern because it may cause death as a result of respiratory failure. Patients in respiratory distress are often intubated with an endotracheal tube so that they can inspire high concentrations of oxygen. Also, if positive-pressure breathing devices are used, the work of breathing deeply is reduced; this can in turn reduce the exhaustion of a seriously ill patient. The gram-negative bacterium *Pseudomonas* is often resistant to multiple antibiotics and is consequently treated with high doses of combined antibiotics.

2. Patients in the final stages of chronic obstructive lung disease are often severely disabled. Minor tasks such as dressing themselves or preparing a simple meal may become major projects. In such a setting, many patients contemplate suicide and some attempt it. Furthermore, this patient's mood may have been affected by his metabolic state.

3. Hypoxia can trigger seizure activity. This patient's dilated pupils indicate that the hypoxia was sufficiently severe to cause a disturbance in brainstem function. The pattern of multiple acute episodes during a relatively short period suggests that the patient could no

87

CASE

three years. The patient had a 30-pack-year smoking history, but had stopped smoking two years previously. He had not had seizures before those described above. Physical examination revealed a comatose patient who was responsive only to deep pain.[4] Breath sounds were clear. Heart sounds were distant. A chest radiograph showed prominent hilar vessels (Fig. 14-1). Arterial blood gases before intubation were pH 7.47 (normal, pH 7.38 to 7.44), PCO_2 58 mmHg (normal, 35 to 45 mmHg), PO_2 58 mmHg (normal, 80 to 100 mmHg). Serum electrolytes were abnormal for sodium (119 mEq/L; normal, 137 to 145 mEq/L) and chloride (74 mEq/L; normal, 94 to 107 mEq/L). The patient was taking a variety of medications including furosemide.[5]

Phenytoin was administered to control his seizures. Lumbar puncture showed a pressure of 350 mm water (normal, <200 mm). The cerebrospinal fluid contained normal protein and glucose levels and no cells. Electrocardiographic studies on the day of admission showed a right bundle branch block, which was unchanged from one year earlier. On the second hospital day, electrocardiographic studies demonstrated anterior and inferior cardiac wall ischemia, with normal serum creatine phosphokinase.[6] Unenhanced computed tomography of the head gave normal results. The patient had a right-sided seizure focus. A neurology consultation obtained on the fifth hospital day demonstrated right hemisphere abnormality. The findings were thought to be most consistent with cortical vein thrombosis, with hyponatremia and dehydration.[7]

Over the next three weeks, the patient experienced waxing and waning mental status with periods of unresponsiveness. He was sometimes somnolent and confused, and sometimes agitated and paranoid. His hemoglobin levels decreased steadily from normal (13.3 to 17.7 g/100 ml) to 8.8 g/100 ml. Arterial blood gases, on 30% O_2 by face mask, were pH 7.29, PCO_2 72 mmHg, and PO_2 36 mmHg. Several hours after the final blood gas studies, the patient was found unresponsive with profound hypotension. He died one hour later, 24 days after admission.[8]

Autopsy revealed widespread evidence of

DISCUSSION

longer tolerate even trivial respiratory insults. In retrospect, it might have been prudent to have admitted the patient after his first visit to the emergency room.

4. It is unfortunately relatively common for patients to give up smoking only when their respiratory disease becomes so severe that they are physically unable to smoke. Coma indicates more serious neurological dysfunction than does seizure activity. Although the patient's respiratory state is an obvious possible cause of coma, other causes or contributing factors should also be considered. Causes that should at least be briefly considered include renal or hepatic dysfunction, previously undiagnosed diabetes leading to diabetic coma, cerebral hemorrhage, and electrolyte disturbances. Given the patient's history of attempted suicide, poisoning or drug overdose is also possible.

5. The patient's high PCO_2 and low PO_2 suggest that he was in chronic respiratory acidosis. However, the pH of the blood was higher than normal, suggesting that the patient was also experiencing metabolic alkalosis. One of the most common reasons for developing metabolic alkalosis is excessive loss of chloride ions secondary to vomiting or to use of diuretics. This patient was not vomiting, but he was on the potent diuretic furosemide for cor pulmonale. Serum chloride levels were abnormally low. Both hyponatremia and alkalosis can cause seizures and coma. The patient's hyponatremia may also be the result of excessive diuresis. Arterial blood gases before intubation were not as severely abnormal as might have been expected from his symptoms. This is probably a reflection of the general principle that a combination of metabolic insults often produces much more severe damage than each insult might individually produce.

6. Phenytoin can effectively control seizures with many causes. The increased intracranial pressure in this patient may have been due to central nervous system edema secondary to injury. If myocardial infarction was occurring, serum creatine phosphokinase levels would have been higher.

7. The patient's seizures continued, and neurological examination demonstrated right hemisphere pathology. The right hemisphere damage may have contributed to his prominent neuropsychiatric symptoms. It is probable that his hypoxia and metabolic state were sufficient to cause the neurological damage.

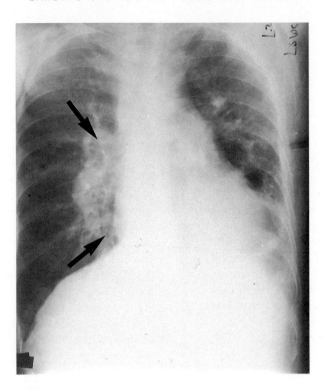

Fig. 14-1. The hilar vessels *(arrows)* in this chest radiograph are prominent, reflecting the enlargement of the main branches of the pulmonary arteries seen in pulmonary hypertension.

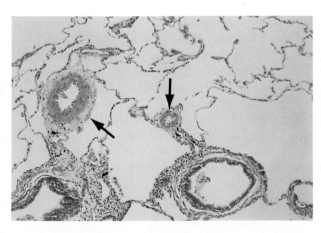

Fig. 14-2. Pulmonary hypertension (high power photomicrograph, hematoxylin and eosin). Two small arteries are visible *(arrows)*. Both of these small arteries resemble small arteries in the systemic circulation and have much thicker muscle layers than are usually present in small pulmonary arteries. Such thickened arterial walls can occur in chronic pulmonary hypertension. Enlarged alveoli, suggesting emphysema, can also be seen.

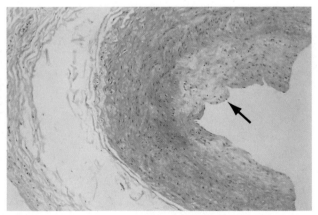

Fig. 14-3. Pulmonary atherosclerosis (low power photomicrograph, hematoxylin and eosin). The section shown is from a branch of a main pulmonary artery. The intima *(arrow)* is markedly thickened, so that the artery resembles a medium-sized atherosclerotic artery from the systemic system. Atherosclerosis involving the pulmonary system is common in patients with pulmonary hypertension.

CASE

chronic obstructive pulmonary disease that included subpleural bullous emphysema, chronic bronchitis, and bronchiectasis (Fig. 14-2). Modest pleural effusions were present, as were bilateral pleural adhesions. Pulmonary atherosclerosis was present (Fig. 14-3).[9] The heart showed right ventricular hypertrophy and cardiomegaly consistent with cor pulmonale. The spleen and liver were congested. The kidneys were edematous. The brain was also edematous (weight, 1,600 g) and was submitted for neuropathological examination. It appeared to have gross evidence of encephalomalacia in the right frontal cortex, but this impression was not confirmed microscopically. No evidence of cortical vein thrombosis was found. Death was considered to be secondary to respiratory failure.[10]

DISCUSSION

8. Although the patient's central nervous system was most obviously affected, there is clinical and anatomical evidence that, as is typical when disease compromises a physiological function necessary to many tissues, many other systems were also involved. The patient had cor pulmonale, and there was electrocardiographic evidence of ischemia (probably actually hypoxia) during his time in hospital. The terminal hypotension may have been a consequence of inadequate pumping by the heart. The patient also had a slowly dropping hematocrit during his terminal illness. This may have reflected a failure of synthesis by the bone marrow as a result of his disturbed metabolic state. The patient's liver and spleen were found to be congested at autopsy, reflecting increased venous pressures produced by the failing right side of the heart. The kidneys, although not obviously diseased clinically, were found at autopsy to be edematous, probably reflecting hypoxic and metabolic damage.

9. The patient's lungs showed changes at autopsy that can be attributed to his chronic lung disease. The phrase *subpleural bullous emphysema* refers to the presence of macroscopic air spaces in the outer regions of the lung, directly beneath the pleural surface. Bronchiectasis is characterized by chronic dilation of bronchi and bronchioles. Pleural effusions are accumulations of fluid in the pleural space and often reflect inflammation of the pleura. Pleural adhesions are scar tissue attaching the pleura to the lung and were probably caused by the patient's earlier episodes of pneumonia.

10. Cortical vein thrombosis was considered to be a possible cause, but this hypothesis was not substantiated at autopsy. Encephalomalacia (softening of the brain) is often the result of metabolic, ischemic, or hypoxic damage.

Chronic Obstructive Pulmonary Disease

Tobacco smoke produces chronic bronchitis, with replacement of the vulnerable ciliated columnar epithelium by sturdier squamous epithelium. The irritation also causes increased sputum production by an increased number of bronchial goblet cells, and enlarged mucous glands cause increased sputum production. Sputum tends to collect in the airways and may occlude the lumena of bronchi and bronchioles. Tobacco smoke also causes emphysema by inducing an inflammatory reaction composed predominantly of neutrophils that release a serine elastase which damages the elastic tissue of the lungs. The elastase activity is inhibited in normal lungs by the proteolytic enzyme α_1-antitrypsin. Tobacco smoke, however, inactivates the α_1-antitrypsin and allows digestion of the elastic tissue of the lungs to continue. The damaged alveoli are then vulnerable to rupture during breathing and coughing.

Although both chronic bronchitis and emphysema occur in smokers, patients vary in the degree to which one or the other process dominates the clinical picture. In patients with emphysema, both air spaces and blood vessels are lost and little perfusion-ventilation mismatch occurs. The patient maintains adequate blood oxygenation and low carbon dioxide levels until late in the disease by chronic hyperventilation. The adequate levels of oxygenation also tend to prevent pulmonary hypertension and right-sided heart failure, although these conditions may develop in a few patients with advanced disease. Physically, the patient with predominant emphysema tends to have a barrel chest, a rosy face, and little edema.

In contrast, patients with chronic bronchitis characteristically cough a great deal, both from irritation of the airways by the original irritant and as a method of improving removal of sometimes copious quantities of sputum. Significant perfusion-ventilation mismatch occurs since ventilation of alveoli is blocked but blood flow remains intact. The patient is typically cyanotic since he has effectively developed a large shunt through the lungs, where oxygenation of the blood and removal of carbon dioxide does not occur. The lower arterial oxygen tension predisposes the patient to pulmonary hypertension, leading to cor pulmonale and thence to edema.

Questions

1. What pulmonary problems did this patient have? What was their cause? How did his respiratory disease affect his heart?
2. How did this patient's progressively worsening pulmonary disease affect his life? What would you try to do to help a patient such as this one?
3. How did the patient's neurological status change with time? What factors were thought to contribute to his changing neurological status? How did he die? What was found at autopsy?

Selected Reading

MacNee W: Right ventricular function in cor pulmonale. Cardiology 75(suppl. 1):30–40, 1988.

Palevsky HI, Fishman AP: Chronic cor pulmonale. Etiology and management. JAMA 263:2347–2353, 1990.

Snider GL: Chronic obstructive pulmonary disease: risk factors, pathophysiology, and pathogenesis. Annu Rev Med 40:411–429, 1989.

15 DIVERTICULAR DISEASE IN A PATIENT WITH α_1-ANTITRYPSIN DEFICIENCY

Key Words | emphysema, α_1-antitrypsin deficiency, diverticulitis

CASE

The patient was a 77-year-old man with severe emphysema secondary to α_1-antitrypsin deficiency. He also had asthma. He had been treated for several years with steroids and bronchodilators.[1] One brother had severe emphysema. The patient's α_1-antitrypsin level was 29.8 mg/100 ml (normal, 125 to 213 mg/100 ml) six weeks before admission.[2] Three weeks before his death, the patient was admitted to the hospital with nausea, vomiting, weight loss, and fatigue. During that hospitalization, his stool was noted to be positive by the guaiac test for occult blood. A question of a gastrointestinal cancer was raised.[3] Upper gastrointestinal series and panendoscopy gave normal results. A barium enema showed sigmoid and distal descending colon diverticula (Fig. 15-1). A sigmoid constricting lesion was also observed that was considered consistent with neoplasm, diverticulitis, or spasm.[4] Colonoscopy was suboptimal because of the patient's pulmonary status. The distal sigmoid lesion was not evaluated further, because the patient's poor pulmonary status would not permit surgery if cancer was found.[5]

The patient was released from the hospital two and one-half weeks after admission. He was seen in the emergency room four days later for a history of poor oral intake since his release.[6] Physical

DISCUSSION

1. α_1-Antitrypsin is an enzyme that degrades proteolytic enzymes. Adults with α_1-antitrypsin deficiency can develop a severe panlobular emphysema. Steroids minimize inflammation and consequently reduce the release of proteolytic enzymes. Bronchodilators relieve asthma.
2. Many different genetic variants of the α_1-antitrypsin gene have been described. Low levels of serum α_1-antitrypsin are diagnostic.
3. Nausea, vomiting, weight loss, and fatigue are all nonspecific symptoms that raised the possibilities of chronic infection, carcinoma, and gastrointestinal disease. The occult blood in the stool suggested gastrointestinal disease.
4. Diverticula produce a very characteristic picture of multiple contrast-filled outpouchings on barium enema. Although contrast studies can identify regions of the gastrointestinal tract where disease is present, definitive diagnosis of a problem usually requires more invasive procedures that permit biopsy of suspicious lesions.
5. Invasive procedures often require considerable cooperation by the patient. Breathing difficulties, severe pain, or neurological dysfunction may all impair a patient's ability to cooperate with or tolerate invasive procedures.
6. There are multiple reasons for poor oral intake, in-

93

CASE

examination demonstrated a pulse of 145/min (normal, 60 to 100/min) with blood pressure of 60 mmHg/palpable (normal, 100 to 140/60 to 90 mmHg). He appeared to be severely dyspneic. The remainder of the physical examination was not recorded because the patient appeared to be about to suffer cardiopulmonary arrest.[7] The arrest occurred shortly thereafter. He was resuscitated pharmacologically and required subsequent vasopressor support. A spontaneous right-sided tension pneumothorax developed; it was treated by the insertion of an 18-gauge catheter into the right lateral chest wall.[8] During this period the patient also developed an agonal cardiac rhythm, and cardiopulmonary resuscitation was reinitiated. Discussion with the patient's physician about his clinical history and prognosis led to the decision to discontinue cardiopulmonary resuscitation efforts, and the patient was pronounced dead.[9]

At autopsy, a constricting lesion of the distal colon was found, which was due to diverticular disease (Fig. 15-2). The sections of involved colon revealed numerous diverticula, which opened onto a common cavity. Perforation of the acutely and chronically inflamed colonic diverticula resulted in a paracolic abscess cavity that encircled the sigmoid colon. In response to the inflammation, the wall was markedly thickened and the overlying adipose tissue was firm and matted. Both of these processes contributed to the narrowed luminal circumference. Postmortem blood cultures contained the gastrointestinal organisms *Streptococcus faecalis* and *Enterobacter aerogenes*.[10] Bilateral panlobular pulmonary emphysema was noted that was consistent with α_1-antitrypsin deficiency (Fig. 15-3). The liver, although not cirrhotic, did have periodic acid-Schiff–positive hyaline globules, and increased cytoplasmic α_1-antitrypsin staining was seen on immunoperoxidase stain (Fig. 15–4).[11] In summary, the patient suffered from α_1-antitrypsin deficiency with resultant severe pulmonary emphysema and complications of colonic diverticulosis. Terminally, he suffered from acute diverticulitis with resultant septicemia.

DISCUSSION

cluding difficulty in chewing or swallowing, fatigue or depression, dementia or delirium, and pain or nausea. When a patient such as this one is interviewed, more information should be obtained about the specific reasons why the oral intake was poor.

7. High pulse rate and low blood pressure suggest developing cardiopulmonary arrest. Hemorrhage, myocardial infarction, and sepsis should have been considered as possible causes in this patient. Given his known severe emphysema and asthma, his respiratory distress may have represented merely a modest worsening of existing lung disease that was just sufficient to cause him to be severely dyspneic at rest. Alternatively, another process, such as pneumonia or pulmonary edema, may have intervened.

8. Spontaneous pneumothorax occurs when an emphysematous bleb near the pleural surface ruptures and permits air to enter the pleural space, causing partial or complete collapse of the adjacent lung. The diagnosis is clinically suspected by the sudden onset of severe dyspnea or a sudden worsening of dyspnea. Pneumothorax is more likely to occur in a patient in respiratory distress who is inhaling violently or in a patient being artificially resuscitated by either vigorous mouth-to-mouth resuscitation or positive-pressure mechanically assisted breathing. The insertion of an 18-gauge needle is an emergency maneuver that can be quickly performed and will often relieve the pneumothorax by permitting the trapped air to be expelled through the needle's lumen.

9. The dying myocardium produces an erratic rhythm with markedly distorted QRS complexes of various shapes. The presence of indicators of severe damage to the heart, such as the agonal rhythm, suggests that severe damage to other organs, including the brain, lungs, and kidneys, may have also occurred. Although such damage was not explicitly stated in the patient's clinical record, the awareness of the high probability that it had occurred in this already fragile patient may have contributed to the decision to discontinue resuscitative efforts.

10. Although diverticular disease is often asymptomatic, complications such as acute or chronic infection may occur. In this patient, inflammation of diverticula progressed to formation of an abscess, which in turn

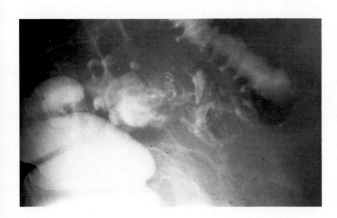

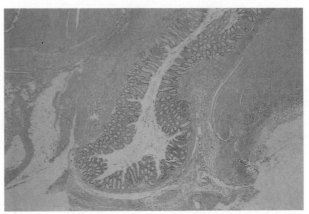

Fig. 15-1. Diverticulosis demonstrated by barium enema. Multiple diverticuli are visible as small outpouchings in the descending *(above right)* and sigmoid *(middle)* colon.

Fig. 15-2. Diverticulosis (low power photomicrograph, hematoxylin and eosin, from another case). The majority of the intestinal lumen lies above the field. The mucosa *(center field)* has completely penetrated the muscle layers *(right* and *left)* of the intestine. Peritonitis can complicate diverticulitis, since an abscess involving the deepest regions of a diverticulum may have only a short distance to penetrate before breaking into the peritoneal cavity.

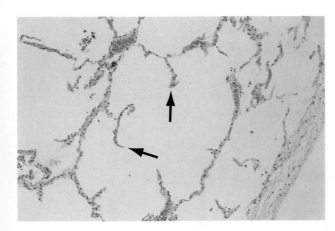

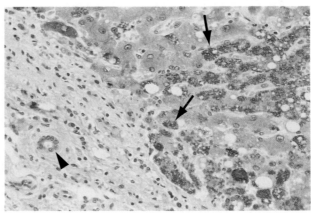

Fig. 15-3. Emphysema in α_1-antitrypsin deficiency (low power photomicrograph, hematoxylin and eosin). Enlarged alveoli are present around the edges of the field. The alveolar walls are relatively avascular. A terminal bronchiole is present in center field and is recognizable by the multiple free alveolar walls *(arrows)* protruding into the lumen. Emphysema caused by α_1-antitrypsin deficiency characteristically produces a panlobular pattern, which is more easily identified on gross than on microscopic specimens.

Fig. 15-4. Liver involvement in α_1-antitrypsin deficiency (high power photomicrograph, immunological stain for α_1-antitrypsin). As discussed in the text, α_1-antitrypsin deficiency is a deficiency of α_1-antitrypsin secretion into the blood. However, α_1-antitrypsin, or perhaps its immunologically equivalent precursor, continues to be synthesized by liver cells. In this field, intracellular accumulations of the α_1-antitrypsin are visible as dark-brown globules of various sizes *(arrows)*. Also visible is extensive periportal fibrosis *(lower left)*. A bile duct is visible in the fibrosis as a small ring of nuclei surrounding a clear lumen *(arrowhead)*.

DISCUSSION

led to septicemia with resulting cardiovascular collapse and initiated the events that resulted in death. Multiple organisms are typically isolated from infections that are initiated by perforation of the intestines.

11. The defect in α_1-antitrypsin deficiency appears to be one of inadequate release of normal α_1-antitrypsin from the liver in most patients with reduced serum levels. Liver samples from these patients typically show cytoplasm inclusions that stain intensely with the periodic acid-Schiff carbohydrate stain. The intense staining reaction occurs because the protein in the inclusions has covalently bonded sugar molecules. The protein appears immunologically to be either α_1-antitrypsin or a closely related compound. The inclusions appear to be relatively benign in most patients. In others, cirrhosis of the liver may occur in either neonatal or adult life.

α_1-Antitrypsin Deficiency

α_1-Antitrypsin is a serum enzyme that is synthesized by the liver and whose action is to degrade a wide variety of proteases. It is thought that the physiological role of the protein may be to limit the action of proteases released, predominantly by neutrophils and activated macrophages, at sites where inflammation is present. Genetic studies have shown that this enzyme is quite variable, and is encoded by at least 26 codominant alleles, which are designated alphabetically. In one of the resulting phenotypes, produced by the homozygous condition for the Z allele, the serum levels of α_1-antitrypsin are typically only 10 to 15% of the levels present in the common, normal phenotype that is homozygous for the M allele. Certain other homozygous and heterozygous states may also cause sufficiently low serum enzymes to be associated with disease.

Although one would expect many organs to be vulnerable to reduced levels of α_1-antitrypsin, the most serious disease occurs in the lungs, where a severe emphysema can be produced. The mechanism appears to be unopposed proteolysis caused by the release of pro-

teases during inflammation, leading to the destruction of the pulmonary elastic membrane and hence loss of alveolar elasticity and permanent distention of alveoli.

The liver is also vulnerable in α_1-antitrypsin deficiency, although by a different mechanism. Serum deficiency of α_1-antitrypsin appears to be usually related to inadequate release rather than impaired synthesis of the enzyme. The liver cells contain eosinophilic cytoplasmic granules (the enzyme is a glycoprotein) that appear to be immunologically similar or identical to α_1-antitrypsin. In many patients, the accumulation of these granules never appears to cause liver dysfunction or disease. In others, however, a wide variety of hepatic syndromes can be produced. A dangerous hepatitis that affects some newborns may either resolve spontaneously or lead to childhood cirrhosis. Other babies may show only mildly altered liver function tests or no disease at all. In adults, a chronic hepatitis can be produced that resembles chronic hepatitis B infection clinically, but without evidence of viral infection. Although the reason for the clinical heterogeneity of the liver disease is still unknown, it is thought that perhaps the cytoplasmic granules are benign in healthy hepatocytes but may potentiate damage initiated by other, independent factors or events (hepatotoxins, infections, etc.) that are not present in all patients.

Questions

1. What respiratory problems did this patient have? What is the relationship between α_1-antitrypsin and emphysema? How were the patient's respiratory problems treated? How did his respiratory status affect his medical status?
2. What gastrointestinal and systemic symptoms caused this patient to seek medical attention? What were the results of his gastrointestinal studies? Why could a definitive diagnosis not be made? How would you feel about making a decision to not at-tempt further diagnostic or therapeutic procedures in a fragile patient?
3. Why was a complete physical examination not performed when this patient was readmitted? Describe the patient's medical course after readmission. How would you recognize and treat each of his problems? How did he die? What were the autopsy findings?

Selected Readings

Buist AS: Alpha-1-antitrypsin deficiency in lung and liver disease. Hosp Pract (Off) 24:51–59, 1989.

Rege RV, Nahrwold DL: Diverticular disease. Curr Probl Surg 26:133–189, 1989.

Snider GL: Chronic obstructive pulmonary disease: risk factors, pathophysiology, and pathogenesis. Annu Rev Med 40:411–429, 1989.

16 OAT CELL CARCINOMA

Key Words | occult cancer, oat cell carcinoma, metastatic disease

CASE

A 77-year-old man was admitted because of two to three months of increasing abdominal girth and fatigue. Diffuse abdominal pain was present, especially in the right upper quadrant, and was exacerbated on deep inspiration and cough. There was no radiation of the pain.[1] The patient had experienced significantly decreased appetite for the preceding several weeks. A cough with yellow sputum had been present for one week. The patient had peptic ulcer disease, which produced occasional epigastric pain, but for which he had never been hospitalized. He had a 60-pack-year history of smoking cigarettes, but had switched to pipe smoking 20 years before admission. He stopped pipe smoking six weeks before admission. He had been drinking four shots of whiskey per day for many years. Review of systems was notable for chest pain with mild to moderate exertion.[2]

Physical examination revealed a well-developed, elderly man with moderate hypertension. The liver was enlarged, firm, and tender, with guarding present on the right side. A firm, mobile, nontender lymph node was present in the inguinal area. Results of a rectal examination were positive for occult blood. The prostate was enlarged, firm, nontender, and smooth. A chest radiograph taken on admission showed a lobulated appearance in the inferior aspect of the right hilum, suggesting a focal mass lesion.[3] The impression was either colonic or lung carcinoma with liver metastases.

Computed tomography of the abdomen showed an enlarged inhomogeneous liver with inhomogeneous enhancing characteristics. No ev-

DISCUSSION

1. Increasing abdominal girth suggest ascites or tumor. Fatigue may have many causes, including renal or hepatic dysfunction, pulmonary or cardiac disease, and tumor. Diffuse abdominal pain suggests gastrointestinal disease that probably involved the liver or gallbladder, since the pain was most prominent in the right upper quadrant. Exacerbation of the pain with deep inspiration and cough would be consistent with involvement of the liver or diaphragm, since these are moved during inspiration. The absence of radiation of the pain suggested that the stomach, duodenum, and pancreas were not involved.

2. Decreased appetite suggests cancer or gastrointestinal obstruction. One week of productive cough suggests bronchopneumonia, which may or may not have been related to the patient's abdominal complaints. A history of peptic ulcer disease, smoking, and alcohol use raised the possibilities of gastric carcinoma, bronchogenic carcinoma, and cirrhosis. The chest pain may have been angina.

3. An enlarged and tender liver confirmed the presence of liver disease. A palpable lymph node in the inguinal area suggested the possibility of metastatic cancer, possibly prostatic cancer. Occult blood in the stool raised the possibility of a gastrointestinal origin of the cancer. Alternatively, the patient's peptic ulcer may have been bleeding. An enlarged, firm, smooth prostate in an elderly man is probably benign prostatic hypertrophy. A focal mass lesion near the hilum of the lung suggested that a process such as tumor or granulomatous disease was present in the hilum or mediastinal nodes.

4. The computed tomogram and special studies tended to support a diagnosis of metastatic cancer. The absence of evidence of gastrointestinal neoplasm, cou-

99

CASE

idence of neoplasm was apparent on barium enema. Computed tomography of the chest revealed a right hilar mass. Also noted were right pleural effusion and ascites. Postobstructive consolidation or extension of the tumor involved the posterior portion of the right upper lobe.[4] There was also extension and/or lymphadenopathy involving the subcarinal, pretracheal, and periesophageal areas. A liver biopsy showed undifferentiated carcinoma, which was thought to probably be metastatic disease. Upper gastrointestinal studies showed areas of active ulceration in the duodenal bulb, which might have been the origin of the occult blood in the stool.[5]

It proved difficult to find evidence of tumor in the lung. The right upper lobe bronchus showed erythema and narrowing of all three bronchial segments, but no intrabronchial lesions were present. Bronchial washing and brushing showed no evidence of cancer. One sputum sample showed atypical squamous epithelial cells. Cultures of sputum samples taken at different times during the two weeks after admission contained *Streptococcus viridans, Neisseria flava*, nonhemolytic *Streptococcus, Klebsiella*, and *Candida tropicalis*. The bronchial washing did not contain *Legionella* or acid-fast bacteria.[6]

After the above studies, the patient was thought to have undifferentiated metastatic carcinoma to the liver. The site of origin was thought to be the lung, despite the negative bronchoscopy and cytology results. A decision to avoid extraordinary measures was made after a discussion between the attending physician, the family members, and the patient.[7] The plan was to send the patient to a hospice. However, approximately two weeks after admission, the patient became more lethargic and later became obtunded. His condition rapidly deteriorated, and he was found dead several days later.[8]

At autopsy, extensive tumor involvement of the right upper lobe near the hilum was found. Metastases were present in the pleura, right lower lobe, hilar nodes, mediastinal nodes, abdominal nodes, liver, and bone (Figs. 16-1 to 16-3). The

DISCUSSION

pled with the pulmonary and mediastinal findings, suggested lung rather than colonic cancer.
5. This pattern of lymph node involvement would be typical of lung cancer since the lymphatic drainage of the lungs is to the noted lymph nodes. If a tumor is sufficiently poorly differentiated, the site of origin may not be recognizable in biopsy sections. The duodenal ulceration noted is due to the patient's peptic ulcer disease rather than to a tumor. Primary duodenal cancers are very rare.
6. The combination of bronchoscopy and bronchial washing results is usually, but not always, diagnostic. Difficulty in demonstrating a tumor in the lungs does not disprove its existence. Pneumonia may complicate both primary and metastatic tumor in the lungs. Negative results for *Legionella* and acid-fast bacteria tend to exclude legionellosis and tuberculosis, respectively.
7. Evidence of pulmonary primary tumor included the extensive presumptive involvement of lungs, pleura, and mediastinal nodes, coupled with minimal abdominal involvement with the exception of the liver. Disseminated lung cancer is very difficult to treat because it is not responsive to most chemotherapeutic agents. Consequently, the decision not to treat the patient's cancer was reasonable.
8. The patient's alterations in consciousness may have been due to inadequate pulmonary function as the lungs became progressively involved with tumor, possibly accompanied by pneumonia and pulmonary edema.
9. The extensive involvement of nodes and organs confirm the premortem findings by computed tomography. Determination of the site of origin of a tumor is often easier at autopsy than by biopsy. The samples taken at autopsy are much larger than biopsy samples, and there is consequently an increased chance that either a distinctive microscopic field will be found or special histological studies will better define the tissue of origin. One indication of the rapidity with which lung cancers can spread is that, despite the earlier negative bronchoscopy results, the autopsy showed obstruction of the bronchi only two weeks after the patient's admission.
10. Since staphylococci were not found at admission,

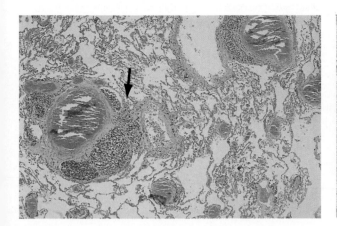

Fig. 16-1. Oat cell carcinoma (low power photomicrograph, hematoxylin and eosin). The cancer is visible as clusters of dark-blue-stained nuclei. It spreads through the lung via the lymphatic channels that follow the arterial supply. Consequently, the heaviest deposition of tumor is found around the edges of blood vessels. Tumor can be seen *(arrow)* breaking out of the lymphatic channels to invade the surrounding lung parenchyma.

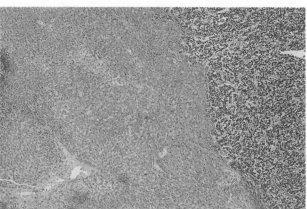

Fig. 16-2. Oat cell carcinoma involving the liver (low power photomicrograph, hematoxylin and eosin). At low power, the tumor nodule *(right)* appears clearly demarcated from the liver *(left)*. The liver shows pale areas of hepatocellular damage, which are probably related to a combination of pressure effects and obstruction of intrahepatic biliary drainage.

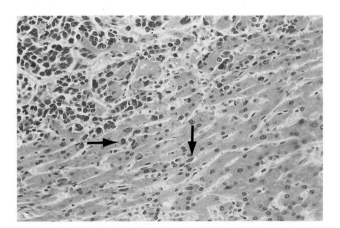

Fig. 16-3. Detail of tumor edge (high power photomicrograph, hematoxylin and eosin). The higher power shows that the edge of the tumor in the liver is poorly defined. Isolated tumor cells *(arrows)* can be recognized separating hepatocytes and invading deep into the adjacent parenchyma. Few or no inflammatory cells are present, suggesting that the patient's cellular immune system is not involved in limiting the spread of the tumor.

CASE

histological diagnosis was small-cell anaplastic carcinoma, also known as *oat cell carcinoma*. By the time of death, the tumor in the right upper lobe had obstructed the bronchi.[9] A focal bronchopneumonia, found at postmortem culture to be caused by coagulase-positive staphylococci, also involved the right upper lobe. Intrahepatic cholestasis was present secondary to obstruction of intrahepatic bile drainage caused by the metastatic disease. The patient also had evidence of emphysema, coronary artery and aortic atherosclerosis, and chronic peptic ulcer disease. The cause of death was considered to be widely metastatic carcinoma complicated by bronchopneumonia.[10]

DISCUSSION

this bronchopneumonia may represent a new infection. The intrahepatic cholestasis was the probable cause of the patient's "tea-colored" urine noted in the clinical history. This offers presumptive evidence that the liver tumor had been present for at least one year.

Lung Cancer

Lung cancer, and in particular bronchogenic carcinoma, is the most common form of cancer in the United States. Several histological varieties of bronchogenic carcinoma are recognized. The most common are squamous cell carcinoma, small-cell anaplastic (oat cell) carcinoma, and large-cell anaplastic carcinoma. The lesions usually start as a roughened area on the bronchial mucosa that is prone to ulcerate. The right bronchus or its main branches are the most common sites of origin.

Lung cancers are prone to metastasis by several mechanisms. The cancers can fill alveoli and can pass through the pores of Kohn from one alveolus to another. Lymphatic spread, particularly to the same and/or opposite lung, chest, and abdomen, is common because of the heavy distribution of lung lymphatics. Hematogenous spread also occurs, with common metastatic sites being liver, adrenal gland, bones, brain, and kidneys. Direct spread outside the lung can occur. Structures typically involved include the other bronchus and lung, the pleura (resulting in hemorrhagic effusion), and the pericardium and heart. The great vessels can become encircled by tumorous growth. This can lead to constriction of the vena cava, with impaired right atrial filling and to impaired pulmonary circulation or return. The aorta is usually relatively spared because of its thick wall and high blood pressure. Infection may complicate lung cancer, leading to recurring attacks of pneumonia and also possibly to bronchiectasis, abscess, or gangrene. Paralysis of the vocal cords may indicate recurrent laryngeal nerve damage. Paralysis of the diaphragm may indicate phrenic nerve damage. Disruption of autonomic control of thoracic organs is produced by involvement of the vagus nerve. Horner syndrome, with ptosis of the eyelid, small pupil, and ipsilateral absence of sweating, is produced by involvement of the sympathetic system. Severe hemorrhage occasionally results from the invasion of a large vessel in the wall of a bronchus.

In addition to damage caused by metastatic cancer, lung cancers can produce a variety of effects on distant tissues. These paraneoplastic syndromes are often related to tumor products with endocrine or metabolic effects. Oat cell lung cancers are particularly likely to produce paraneoplastic syndromes. Syndromes produced include secretion of antidiuretic hormone leading to the development of hyponatremia, and secretion of adrenocorticotropic hormone (ACTH), leading to Cushing syndrome. Ectopic parathyroid production by epidermoid cancers can cause hypercalcemia and hypophosphatemia. Epidermoid cancers can also cause skeletal connective tissue syndromes such as digital clubbing and hypertrophic pulmonary osteoarthritis. Disturbances in the blood coagulation system can produce disseminated intravascular coagulation and nonbacterial thrombotic endocarditis. Effects on neurological and muscular systems may include degeneration of the cerebellum or cortex, peripheral neuropathies, polymyositis, and a syndrome called the Eaton-Lambert syndrome, which resembles myasthenia gravis.

Questions

1. With what symptoms did this patient present? Disease of which organ systems was suggested by his history and symptoms? Which of his medical problems might have been interrelated?
2. What was observed on physical examination of this patient? What did laboratory and radiological studies show? What findings suggested that this patient had metastatic disease?

3. Which tissues were considered possible sources of the patient's primary tumor? Why is it important to try to identify the primary tumor when a patient has widely metastatic disease? What studies were undertaken to demonstrate the patient's primary tumor? How successful was the attempt to identify the primary tumor? How did the patient die? What was found at autopsy?

Selected Reading

Drings P: Preoperative assessment of lung cancer. Chest 96(suppl. 1):42s–44s, 1989.

Goodman GE, Livingston RB: Small cell lung cancer. Curr Probl Cancer 13:1–54, 1989.

Nicolson GL: Cancer metastasis: tumor cell and host organ properties important in metastasis to specific secondary sites. Biochim Biophys Acta 948:175–224, 1988.

GASTROINTESTINAL TRACT

17 SQUAMOUS CELL CARCINOMA OF THE ESOPHAGUS

Key Words | esophageal cancer, metastatic disease, pneumonia

CASE

A 52-year-old woman presented to a physician with a 25-lb (11.4 kg) weight loss during the preceding three months. She had experienced increasing difficulty swallowing first solid and then semisolid foods. She had a history of 30 years of heavy cigarette and beer consumption.[1] A barium swallow demonstrated irregular luminal narrowing of the mid-esophagus (Fig. 17-1). Endoscopic biopsy of the lesion showed well-differentiated squamous cell carcinoma. The patient then underwent a total esophagectomy with cervical esophagogastric anastomosis.[2] It was noted during surgery that the tumor was adherent to the prevertebral fascia. Pathological examination of the esophagus showed that the tumor involved the complete thickness of the specimen. After surgery, the patient experienced persistent back and upper extremity pain. She was treated with radiation therapy to the chest and back for the next month.[3]

The patient was readmitted three months after surgery with severe back, chest, and upper extremity pain. She was also having increasing difficulty in eating. Her oral intake for the three days preceding admission had consisted of one to two bottles of soft drinks per day. She had lost approximately 11 lb (5.0 kg) in the two weeks before admission.[4] Pertinent physical and laboratory findings included stool positive by the guaiac test,

DISCUSSION

1. The combination of weight loss and difficulty in swallowing raised the possibility of oral or esophageal cancer. Alternatively, the weight loss may not have been due to tumor, but instead may have been related to inadequate nutrition secondary to difficulty with swallowing. If this were the case, other processes that can involve the esophagus, such as systemic sclerosis or motility disorders, should have been considered. Alcohol and cigarette smoke both chronically irritate the esophageal mucosa and are consequently risk factors for the development of esophageal cancer.

2. A barium swallow is often the first diagnostic test performed in patients with swallowing disorders. It can demonstrate motility disorders, constriction, and outpouchings in the esophagus. Irregular luminal narrowing suggests strictures or infiltration of the esophagus by tumor. The mid-esophagus is a common site for squamous carcinoma of the esophagus. Biopsy of the lesion is necessary to confirm the diagnosis. In total esophagectomy, the diseased portion of the esophagus is resected with wide margins. The stomach is then brought into the thoracic cavity. Finally, an anastomosis is created between the stomach and the remaining esophagus.

3. Dissemination of the cancer was indicated by involvement of the complete thickness of the esophagus and adherence to the prevertebral fascia. Pain in the thoracic cavity tends to be referred to the back

CASE

anemia, dehydration, and sinus tachycardia with a resting heart rate of 106/min (normal, 60 to 100/min). A chest radiograph showed an infiltrate or atelectasis in the right upper lobe. There was also pneumonitis or edema scattered throughout the lower lobes.[5]

Tube feedings and gentle rehydration were initiated. Methadone was given to relieve pain. Computed tomography of the chest and abdomen revealed probable obstruction of the stomach, bilateral pleural effusions, and a probable right lower lobe infiltrate. There was possible adenopathy from the neck to the abdomen.[6] Several days after admission, the patient began aspirating swallowed fluids (including a barium swallow) and gastric contents. This increased concern that she might develop pneumonia. One week after admission, 20 ml of an amber, translucent fluid was removed by left thoracocentesis. The fluid was

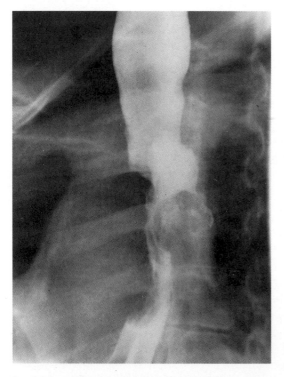

Fig. 17-1. Upper gastrointestinal series shows narrowing of the esophageal lumen by what was found at surgery to be squamous carcinoma of the esophagus.

DISCUSSION

and the upper extremities. Pain after major surgery is common and can be difficult to interpret. The surgery itself can cause pain that takes weeks to months to resolve. Radiation therapy may cause tissue damage or inflammation. Nodules of tumor can compress nerves. Alternatively, inflammation or infection may involve thoracic structures.

4. This patient's persistent pain and difficulty in eating suggest that a tumor may have been obstructing the gastrointestinal tract.

5. The combination of anemia and occult blood in the stool suggest slow, steady oozing of blood from either incisions or cancer. Sinus tachycardia was probably due to the combination of anemia and dehydration. The results of the chest radiograph suggest that the patient may have had pneumonia, invasion of cancer into the bronchi and lungs, or both.

6. It is important not to rehydrate a patient too rapidly as a rapid infusion of fluids may lead to hemodilution, exacerbating the anemia, and may also produce tissue edema as fluid is shifted from the vascular to the extravascular spaces. Methadone is a narcotic similar to morphine. Tumor involvement of pleura can cause pleural effusions. Adenopathy may be caused by tumor involvement of lymph nodes.

7. For many reasons, this patient was at serious risk for the development of pneumonia. Surgery left her vulnerable to aspiration of gastric contents by shortening the esophagus and impairing the patency of the gastroesophageal sphincter. Also, if surgery, endoscopy, and/or tumor invasion have damaged the lower oropharynx, swallowing reflexes may be poorly coordinated. The patient may consequently be vulnerable to aspirating saliva. The presence of stomach in the chest cavity may put pressure on bronchi or lung parenchyma and predispose to partial airway obstruction, another risk factor for pneumonia. Finally, both radiation therapy and metastatic tumor can cause inflammation, leaving the lungs vulnerable to infection. The pneumonia that develops in this setting may be very difficult to treat effectively since multiple organisms may be involved. Thoracocentesis involves inserting a needle through the skin and muscle between the lower ribs to withdraw fluid accumulating in the pleural space. Sterile, translucent fluid without malignant cells suggest that the pleural effusion was a transudate rather than an exudate.

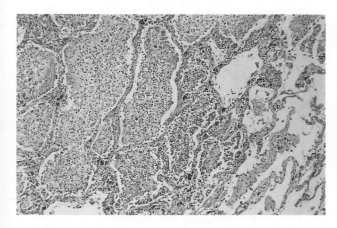

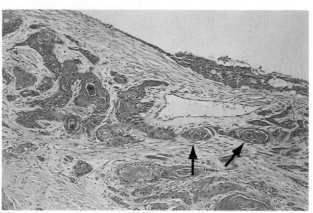

Fig. 17-2. Pneumonia (low power photomicrograph, hematoxylin and eosin). *Pseudomonas aeruginosa* was found in a culture of a specimen of this lung at autopsy. Many alveoli are completely filled with alveolar cells, proteinaceous debris, bacteria, and neutrophils.

Fig. 17-3. Esophageal cancer involving the diaphragm (low power photomicrograph, hematoxylin and eosin). Nests of squamous carcinoma cells are embedded in the fibrous tissue of the diaphragm. Keratin pearls *(arrows),* in which groups of cancer cells mature sufficiently to produce keratin and to mimic normal squamous epithelium, are also apparent.

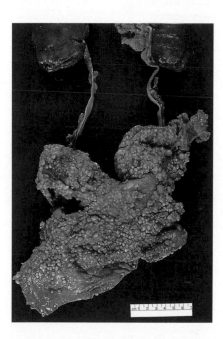

Fig. 17-4. Carcinoma involving the bladder (gross photograph). The surface of the bladder *(below)* and ureters is covered with tumor nodules. The tumor selectively involved the peritoneal covering of the bladder, and the bladder muscle was almost completely free of tumor.

CASE

sterile and contained no malignant cells. A sputum sample taken at the same time grew *Pseudomonas aeruginosa* and coagulase-positive and coagulase-negative staphylococci on culture. Therapy with the broad-spectrum antibiotic chloramphenicol was begun.[7]

Two days later, her glottic closure was surgically improved, with good results. She was transferred the next day to a surgical intensive care unit, where she was intubated because of increasing respiratory distress. A tracheostomy was performed the following day. The patient did poorly, with unsuccessful weaning from the ventilator.[8] Gentamicin and tobramycin were added to the antibiotic regimen. Additional sputum cultures were positive for *Candida albicans* and a highly resistant coagulase-positive staphylococcus. Cefoxitin was added to the regimen. A chest radiograph two weeks after admission showed progressive parenchymal consolidation. An epidural catheter was placed for morphine injections to improve pain control. The patient continued to show no clinical improvement for the next three weeks. She experienced bradycardia and then became asystolic approximately six weeks after her final admission and four and one-half months after her esophagectomy.[9] She was found at autopsy to have bronchopneumonia due to *Pseudomonas aeruginosa* (Fig. 17-2). Very extensive metastases were present within the pleural and peritoneal cavities (Figs. 17-3 and 17-4).[10]

DISCUSSION

8. Improving glottic closure reduces the risk of aspiration, but may cause respiratory difficulties by partially occluding the open airways. Since the tracheostomy bypasses the vocal cords and glottis, tracheostomy was expected to restore the patient's respiratory function. Since the tracheostomy did not restore function sufficiently to permit her to be weaned from the ventilatory support, other processes, such as the pneumonia, tumor, and intrathoracic stomach mentioned earlier, probably were major contributors to her respiratory insufficiency.

9. As each new guess about a possible cause of infection was made, another powerful antibiotic was added to the therapy. Despite vigorous therapy, the patient still died of an infection that was not definitively identified until autopsy. Progressive parenchymal consolidation indicates that tumor and pneumonia involvement of the lung was progressing. An epidural catheter can improve pain control by providing high morphine concentrations around spinal nerve roots and the spinal cord. The bradycardia and asystole experienced terminally by this patient were probably the result of impaired brainstem or cardiac function as a result of hypoxia.

10. The finding of *Pseudomonas* at autopsy does not necessarily imply that the antibiotic therapy was inappropriate. The patient may have been infected originally with multiple organisms, of which only the *Pseudomonas*, which is often drug-resistant, survived. Dissemination of the squamous cell carcinoma in the peritoneal cavity is unusual. It occurred in this patient by direct extension.

Esophageal Cancer

Predisposing factors for cancer of the esophagus include many causes of chronic irritation to the esophageal mucosa. Chronic alcohol use and smoking are notable culprits. Achalasia, in which the esophagus fails to contract normally during swallowing, is a predisposing factor because food retained in the esophagus may irritate the mucosa. Caustic substances may cause scars and strictures in which cancer sometimes arises. Gastroesophageal reflux may lead to the development of metaplastic columnar epithelium, another predisposing factor for cancer. Patients with Plummer-Vinson syndrome, a rare entity characterized by iron deficiency anemia and webs in the upper esophagus, have a higher incidence of esophageal cancer. Celiac sprue, a chronic diarrheal disease relieved by removal of gluten from the diet, is also associated with increased incidence.

Esophageal cancer has a very poor prognosis, with one year survival rates of less than 20% and five year survival rates of less than 5%. Radiation therapy, as in this case, is often unsuccessful in limiting the spread of the cancer. The tumor tends to spread by direct extension into a variety of adjacent structures, possibly because the esophagus does not have a serosal surface. Periesophageal spread may be suggested clinically by the presence of steady substernal pain radiating to the back. Erosion into the aorta may result in rapid exsanguination. Involvement of the recurrent laryngeal nerve may cause hoarseness. Fistulas may form between the esophagus and bronchi or pleura and may cause recurrent abscesses or pneumonia.

Questions

1. How did this patient present? How was esophageal cancer diagnosed? What risk factors for development of esophageal cancer did this patient have? What is the prognosis for esophageal cancer? Why is it so serious?

2. Describe this patient's surgery. Where was her stomach after the surgery? What was the significance of the full-thickness involvement of the esophageal wall? What was the purpose of radiation therapy?

3. What types of complications can esophageal cancer cause? What complications did this patient experience? Describe her hospital course. How did she die? What was found at autopsy?

Selected Reading

Ahmed ME, Gustavsson S: Current palliative modalities for esophageal carcinoma. Clinical review. Acta Chir Scand 156:95–98, 1990.

Demeester TR, Barlow AP: Surgery and current management for cancer of the esophagus and cardia. Curr Probl Surg 25:477–605, 1988.

Gelfand MD, Botoman VA: Esophageal motility disorders: a clinical overview. Am J Gastroenterol 82:181–187, 1987.

18 BLEEDING DUODENAL ULCER IN A PATIENT WITH TEMPORAL ARTERITIS

Key Words | temporal arteritis, peptic ulcer, gastrointestinal hemorrhage

CASE

A 69-year-old man developed recurrent bilateral headaches; on physical examination, easily palpable, nodular, temporal arteries were noted. Temporal arteritis was diagnosed (Fig. 18-2). The patient was treated with prednisone, which markedly alleviated his headaches.[1]

Ten months later, the patient developed severe burning epigastric pain. The pain occurred several hours after meals and was relieved by food and antacids. Stools tested positive by the guaiac test for occult blood, and the patient had a mild hypochromic, microcytic anemia.[2] He had a 20-pack-year smoking history. Barium examination of the upper gastrointestinal tract revealed a duodenal ulcer near the pyloric junction (Fig. 18-1). This was treated with antacids, the antihistamine ranitidine, and a lowered prednisone dose.[3]

Colonic polyps and diverticulosis were found on barium enema during evaluation of the ulcer. The patient was admitted six weeks later for removal of the polyps. Physical examination at the time of admission demonstrated mild respiratory distress and some evidence of oral candidiasis, and stools were positive by the guaiac test.[4]

On the second hospital day, before surgical removal of the polyps, the patient abruptly became diaphoretic and was noted to have a drop in

DISCUSSION

1. Temporal arteritis is a chronic inflammation of branches of the carotid arteries, particularly the temporal arteries. The inflammation is granulomatous and can cause marked luminal narrowing as granuloma replaces the vessel wall. A ring of multinucleated giant cells may mark the location of the degenerated internal elastic membrane. The cause of temporal arteritis is unknown. The disease often manifests as a cluster of fever, anemia, and headaches in an elderly patient. In some patients, muscular aching and joint stiffness are also prominent early symptoms; this has led to the suggestion that temporal arteritis may be related to rheumatoid arthritis. The temporal arteries may be easily palpable and have a nodular structure. The disease must be treated, usually with steroids, because the process can involve the ophthalmic arteries and lead to blindness.

2. Patients who are treated with corticosteroids appear to be at increased risk of developing peptic ulcer disease. The mechanism for this vulnerability is not clearly understood, but may be related to alterations in gastric acid secretion and in the gastric and duodenal mucosa. This patient's pain is typical of the pain associated with a duodenal ulcer. The pain of a gastric ulcer may be similar, but often is not relieved by ingestion of food. The occult blood in the stools and the anemia suggest that the patient may have been

CASE

blood pressure. An upper endoscopy study demonstrated that the duodenal ulcer was bleeding. The hemorrhage responded to gastric suction followed by antacid and ranitidine administration. The patient was transfused 2 units of whole blood.[5] The ulcer was oversewn the next day. Additionally, the vagus nerves were sectioned, and pyloroplasty was performed to prevent delayed gastric emptying following the vagotomy.[6]

The patient remained relatively stable postoperatively for approximately two weeks. He then again abruptly became hypotensive and showed a decline in respiratory status; he was transferred to an intensive care unit, where he was intubated.[7] He was febrile and was found to have an atrial arrhythmia. There was also questionable congestive heart failure. Urine culture revealed *Streptococcus faecalis*, and sepsis was suspected. The patient continued to be febrile and hypotensive and

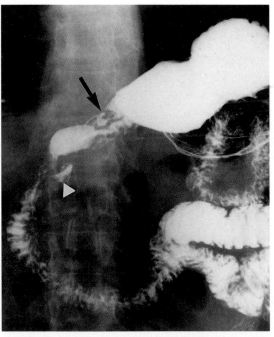

Fig. 18-1. Upper gastrointestinal series with small bowel follow-through shows a duodenal ulcer (arrow). A duodenal diverticulum is also present (arrowhead).

DISCUSSION

bleeding chronically. Hypochromic, microcytic anemia suggests iron deficiency, which is unusual in men who have not been bleeding chronically.

3. Both smoking and corticosteroid use are risk factors for peptic ulcer disease. Most duodenal ulcers (95%) occur within the first portion of the duodenum. They are usually the result of damage to the duodenal mucosa by acid-pepsin secretions from the stomach. Medical therapy of duodenal ulcers is usually directed toward raising the pH of stomach contents. The H_2 receptor antagonists such as cimetidine and ranitidine lower histamine-mediated secretion of hydrochloric acid by parietal cells.

4. It is not uncommon for other conditions, such as the colonic polyps and diverticulosis in this patient, to be found incidentally during the evaluation of an elderly patient. Diverticulosis is characterized by multiple small outpouchings in the colonic wall. Removal of colonic polyps was considered because colonic cancer can develop in polyps. The mild respiratory distress is probably the result of chronic obstructive lung disease secondary to smoking. Persistence of positive stools by the guaiac test suggests that the medical treatment for the ulcer had not been effective. In immunocompromised patients, the fungus *Candida* can invade the oral mucosa. Oral candidiasis, also known as thrush, presents as white mucosal plaques that may be either discrete or confluent.

5. Diaphoresis (especially profuse perspiration) can be caused by massive stimulation of the autonomic nervous system, as occurs in response to suddenly dropping blood pressure. Intense sweating together with dropping blood pressure suggested that this patient had started to bleed severely, probably from the duodenal ulcer. Although some duodenal ulcers heal with medical management, others require surgical management because of recurrent bleeding. Gastric suction will remove most of both the blood and acid in the stomach lumen. Gastric suction is therapeutically important because blood is a notable gastric irritant and its presence might initiate vomiting and because it is easier to rapidly raise the pH of the stomach, and thence the duodenum, if the stomach is empty. Raising the stomach pH will lower the activity of pepsin, which will digest clotted blood at lower pH.

6. Oversewing of the duodenal ulcer was intended to stop the bleeding and protect the injured tissue from

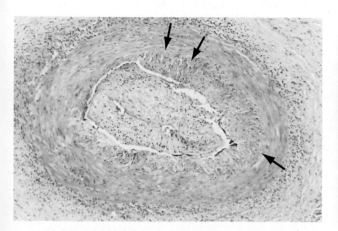

Fig. 18-2. Temporal arteritis (low power photomicrograph, hematoxylin and eosin, from another case). The lumen of the temporal artery is almost completely occluded by fibrotic thickening of the intimal layer. At higher magnification, a few multinucleated giant cells are found in the thickened intima. A lymphocytic infiltration surrounds the artery, and lymphocytes are present in the musculature and intima. The elastic lamina *(arrows)* is partially disrupted.

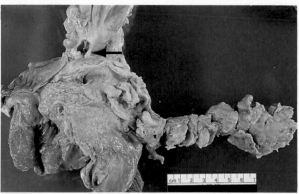

Fig. 18-3. Duodenal ulcer (gross specimen, from another case). The pyloric junction is above; the pancreas is to the right; and the remainder of the duodenum is below. A duodenal ulcer *(arrow)* has completely perforated the duodenum just below the pyloric junction.

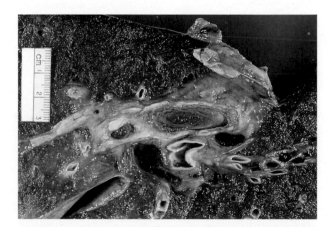

Fig. 18-4. Blood clot in the right main bronchus (gross specimen). A blood clot has completely filled the right main bronchus. This blood was aspirated when the patient vomited after his gastrointestinal tract began to bleed. The aspiration was probably the immediate cause of the patient's death.

CASE

to have poor respiratory status for the next few days; he was then found dead.[8]

At autopsy, massive gastrointestinal hemorrhage was found, the source being the previously oversewn duodenal ulcer (Fig. 18-3). There was acute aspiration of blood, with complete occlusion of the right mainstem bronchus by clot, and bilateral filling of the alveoli with blood (Fig. 18-4). *Candida albicans* was found in cultures of specimens from the peritoneal cavity and from an abscess in the abdominal incision.[9]

DISCUSSION

further damage. Cutting the vagus nerve removed cholinergic stimulation of the gastrointestinal tract and would be expected to consequently reduce gastric secretion. In pyloroplasty, a longitudinal incision is cut through the pylorus and then the incision is resutured transversely, causing an increased effective diameter of the pyloric junction.

7. The surgery clearly did not completely correct the ulcer, as the patient began to bleed again. This episode differs from the previous one in that the patient experienced a sudden decline in respiratory function. One possibility is that this is again an episode of hemorrhage, which in this case has been complicated by aspiration of blood. Alternatively, the patient may have been developing sepsis. The reason for the decline in respiratory function is somewhat unclear. A differential diagnosis including pulmonary edema, pneumonia, worsening chronic obstructive pulmonary disease, and pulmonary embolism would probably have been reasonable.

8. This patient's condition after surgery was poor because he was febrile, had an atrial arrhythmia, and had possible congestive heart failure. Upper urinary tract infections are a common cause of sepsis.

9. The immediate cause of death was apparently aspiration of blood. The patient had an unsuspected abdominal *Candida* infection, probably introduced through the abdominal wound and possibly related to his oral candidiasis, that was not found until autopsy. This infection probably contributed to the patient's poor condition.

Peptic Ulcer

The normal gastric mucosa and proximal duodenal mucosa are very resistant to the corrosive effects of acid-pepsin secretions. However, when the secretions become excessive or when the mucosal resistance is reduced, damage to the mucosa can produce an ulcer. Such an ulcer is characterized by relatively sharp margins and a flat, round to oval base. The depth of the hole varies with the amount of tissue digested. The floor of the hole is invariably smooth and clear as a result of peptic digestion of exudates. If the hole penetrates through the gastric or intestinal wall, perforation occurs. A secondary peritonitis and damage of adjacent organs by acid-pepsin mixtures may follow. Hemorrhage occurs when a vessel in the base of the ulcer is eroded; it is particularly dangerous as it tends to recur as a result of proteolytic digestion of any blood clots that form in the damaged vessel. Chronic peptic ulcers typically produce collagenous scar formation in the adjacent underlying tissue and may cause gastric outlet obstruction due to contraction of the pylorus or first portion of the duodenum.

The pathogenesis of gastric ulcers may be somewhat

different from that of duodenal ulcers. There is evidence that many patients with duodenal ulcers have both enhanced blood gastrin levels after meals and an enhanced gastric acid secretory response to the gastrin. Although acid secretion is necessary for formation of a duodenal ulcer, many patients with gastric ulcer have higher than normal gastric pH. True achlorhydria, however, almost never occurs; if present, it suggests a gastric carcinoma rather than a peptic ulcer. Regurgitation of bile-containing duodenal contents and local ischemia due to vascular disease may be pathogenic factors in some gastric ulcers.

Questions

1. What is temporal arteritis? Why is temporal arteritis considered dangerous and consequently treated aggressively? Why has it been suggested that temporal arteritis may be related to rheumatoid arthritis? How might this patient's temporal arteritis have been related to his peptic ulcer disease?
2. What is the pathophysiology of peptic ulcer development? How was the diagnosis of duodenal ulcer made in this patient? What was found coincidentally during evaluation of this patient's ulcer?
3. How was the ulcer treated? How did the ulcer disease contribute to the patient's death? Describe the patient's hospital course after his elective admission for removal of colonic polyps.

Selected Reading

Friedman G: Peptic ulcer disease. Clin Symp 40:1–32, 1988.

Mehler MF, Rabinowich L: The clinical neuro-ophthalmologic spectrum of temporal arteritis. Am J Med 85:839–844, 1988.

Miller TA: Emergencies in acid-peptic disease. Gastroenterol Clin N Am 17:303–315, 1988.

19 JEJUNAL-ILEAL BYPASS FOR MORBID OBESITY

Key Words | obesity, jejunal-ileal bypass, multiorgan failure

CASE

A 41-year old man was admitted to a hospital because of dehydration and electrolyte disorders. He had been previously admitted on numerous occasions. He had been morbidly obese in his teens and early twenties (maximum weight, 520 lb [235 kg]). When he was 26 years old, he was treated with jejunal-ileal bypass surgery. His weight had decreased to 300 lb (135 kg) over the several years following the surgery. It had again decreased, as a result of a combination of illness and dieting, to 170 lb (77 kg) in his late thirties.[1]

The patient experienced symptoms of short bowel syndrome during the 15 years between the bypass surgery and final admission. The symptoms included chronic diarrhea and, for the year preceding this admission, chronic hypokalemia, hypomagnesemia, and metabolic acidosis. These electrolyte disturbances had been documented in a previous admission as being due to gastrointestinal losses.[2] Three years before this admission, his platelet counts had decreased. A diagnosis of idiopathic thrombocytopenic purpura had been made after demonstration of anti-platelet antibodies in the serum. He had been on long-term prednisone treatment since that time.[3] One year before final admission, he developed symptoms of sepsis and was found to have extensive pelvic-rectal abscesses. He underwent splenectomy one month after release from the hospital for treatment of the

DISCUSSION

1. When dieting measures have been completely unsuccessful and a patient is morbidly obese, surgical shortening of the intestine is sometimes attempted. The operation performed in this patient involved anastomosis of the proximal portion of the jejunum to the terminal portion of the ileum. In this operation, the intervening intestine is not removed, but food preferentially passes through the anastomosis rather than the bypassed intestine. The intent of such surgery is to deliberately produce a syndrome of malabsorption. Ideally, the patient's gastrointestinal function is limited enough to allow substantial weight loss without causing frank malnourishment. In this patient, although the surgery did lead to substantial weight loss, it also led eventually and indirectly to his death.

2. Diarrhea is associated with loss of electrolytes and bases. Consequently, hypokalemia, hypomagnesemia, and metabolic acidosis can occur if a substantial degree of chronic diarrhea is present.

3. Idiopathic thrombocytopenic purpura is characterized by autoimmune destruction of platelets. This leads to seriously reduced platelet counts, with the risk of serious bleeding after minor injury.

4. Long-term treatment with corticosteroids predisposes a patient to opportunistic infection. In this case, the patient developed pelvic-rectal abscesses. Many platelets bound to antibody are removed by the reticuloendothelial system in the spleen. Conse-

119

CASE

abscesses. His prednisone dose was reduced at that time.[4]

One month before his death, the patient was admitted for correction of dehydration, hypomagnesemia, and hypokalemia. The electrolyte abnormalities were promptly corrected.[5] Ultrasonography revealed a fusiform mass in the patient's right lower abdominal quadrant. This mass was considered to be due to a possible intraperitoneal abscess. The patient was treated with antibiotics for two weeks.[6] He complained intermittently of right lower quadrant pain, but was afebrile. The pain was thought to be secondary to erosion of skin since no peritoneal signs were present. His platelet counts were again decreased. Bleeding occurred from intravenous catheter sites, and he had a coagulopathy with prolonged prothrombin and partial thromboplastin times. He was treated with platelet and blood transfusions and broad-spectrum antibiotics.[7]

The patient's general condition continued to deteriorate, with shortness of breath, cough, nausea, and vomiting. A radiograph revealed free air under the diaphragm. Exploratory laparotomy performed 18 days after admission showed intussusception of a portion of the bypassed ileum.[8] One week after surgery, the patient became septic and experienced a decrease in blood pressure that required a pressor agent. Cultures of sputum samples grew *Pseudomonas*. Despite antibiotic treatment, clinical adult respiratory distress syndrome and poor lung function developed. Terminally, he was hypothermic and acidotic. He died two weeks after surgery.[9]

Autopsy results showed diffuse interstitial fibrosis with hyaline membranes and focal acute bronchopneumonia. An abscess with cavitation was present in the right lower lobe (Fig. 19-1). The kidneys microscopically revealed evidence of acute tubular necrosis (Fig. 19-2). Postmortem cultures of blood, urine, and abdominal incision specimens grew *Candida tropicalis*. The proximal jejunum was bypassed to the terminal ileum, and the bypass was intact (Fig. 19-3). The large and small bowels were grossly unremarkable except

DISCUSSION

quently, performing a splenectomy and reducing the patient's prednisone dose appeared to be a reasonable alternative.

5. Correction of dehydration and electrolyte abnormalities involves transfusion with fluids containing appropriately increased concentrations of magnesium and potassium. Such restoration should be done carefully and over a period of several hours, with intermittent monitoring, to reduce the risk of overcorrection.

6. The patient's abdominal mass was misrecognized as an abscess. This illustrates the important clinical point that the patient's history can sometimes be misleading. It is easy to assume that symptoms are due to recurrence of an old problem when actually a new problem has developed. Exacerbation of pain during abdominal examination is an example of a peritoneal sign.

7. The reason for the coagulopathy with prolonged prothrombin and partial thromboplastin times was not completely clear. If the patient was suffering from protein malnourishment as a result of his bypass surgery, his liver may not have been producing adequate quantities of blood-clotting factors. Broad-spectrum antibiotics are useful when infection is suspected, but it has not proved possible to implicate a particular organism.

8. The presence of free air under the diaphragm suggests that perforation of an abdominal structure has occurred. Free air is considered to be a grave finding since the same perforation may permit peritonitis to develop. *Intussusception* refers to the telescoping of one segment of intestine into the lumen of an adjacent segment. It is dangerous because the blood supply to the involved segments may be compromised, possibly leading to death of the involved intestine, and peritonitis as the intestinal wall is digested. The patient's septicemia may have been a result of infection triggered by his intussusception or surgery, or it may have been the consequence of pneumonia.

9. Septicemia can dangerously lower the blood pressure, leading to damage of many organs. *Pseudomonas* was the first organism to be isolated, but was not necessarily the only organism that caused disease in this patient. Many strains of *Pseudomonas* are

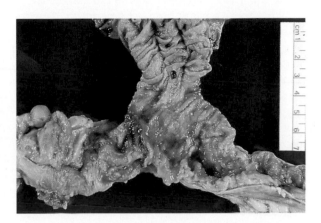

Fig. 19-1. Jejunal-ileal bypass (gross specimen). The proximal jejunum *(above)* is anastomosed to the terminal ileum *(below)*. The patient's anastomosis is patent and has healed well.

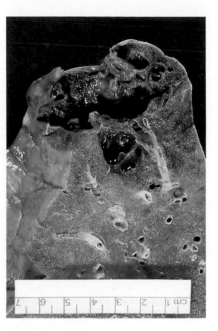

Fig. 19-2. Pulmonary abscess (gross specimen). A large pulmonary abscess with cavitation is present *(above)*. Cavities of this size can be consistently visualized by computed tomography and can often be visualized on chest radiographs.

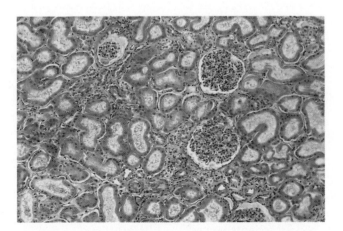

Fig. 19-3. Acute tubular changes (high power photomicrograph, hematoxylin and eosin). The tubules are dilated and contain proteinaceous debris. These changes are commonly observed in mild acute tubular necrosis.

CASE

for fibrous adhesions due to surgery. The cause of death was considered to be respiratory failure secondary to adult respiratory distress syndrome and infection.[10]

DISCUSSION

highly resistant to multiple antibiotics. Other contributing organisms may have been controlled by broad-spectrum antibiotics.

10. The lungs are particularly vulnerable to damage by shock. Acute respiratory distress syndrome is a distinctive syndrome that can develop after hemodynamic shock and can cause death. The lungs may initially appear normal, but over a period of days coagulation, inflammation, and pulmonary edema develop in the injured tissue, producing a characteristic histological picture. The kidneys are also particularly vulnerable and show acute tubular necrosis after ischemic injury. *Candida* infection was clinically unsuspected and was consequently not treated. Fibrous adhesions are bands of connective tissue that form secondary to inappropriate growth of fibroblasts at sites of previous inflammation.

Intestinal Bypass

Diet and exercise programs are preferred measures for control of obesity. Surgical management is usually limited to patients who are at least 100 lb (40 kg) overweight and who have made repeated, well-designed attempts to lose weight by other means. Significant medical or psychological problems that cannot be adequately treated in the presence of continuing obesity are also considered indications.

In intestinal bypass surgery, part of the small intestine is short-circuited. In this case, the beginning portion of the jejunum was connected to the terminal portion of the ileum. Intestinal bypass surgery is usually effective in reducing a patient's weight. Operative and immediate postoperative morbidity and mortality are low. Unfortunately, it is common for patients to experience complications years after the surgery. Loss of electrolytes secondary to intractable diarrhea can disturb electrolyte balance, leading to hypokalemia, hypomagnesemia, and hypocalcemia. Malnutrition with deficiencies in oil-soluble vitamins can occur. These patients are also predisposed to migratory arthralgias and the formation of calcium oxalate kidney stones. Bacterial overgrowth in blind loops can produce intermittent symptoms of fever, pain, obstruction, and abdominal distension. Protein deficiency sometimes causes liver disease which may progress to cirrhosis. Intestinal bypass surgery is now only rarely performed since this broad spectrum of medical complications is considered to limit the usefulness of the procedure. When the operation is used, it is often as a preparative operation, in patients weighing more than 500 lb (200 kg), which is reversed when the patient's weight has been substantially reduced. The definitive operation of gastric restriction is then performed.

Questions

1. Why was this patient treated with jejunal-ileal bypass? How much weight did he lose? What other methods can be used for weight control? What are the advantages and disadvantages of these methods?

2. What complications did this patient experience that were related to his bypass surgery? Propose mechanisms that might produce each of these complications. What is idiopathic thrombocytopenic purpura? How did this disorder and its sequelae complicate the patient's hospital course?

3. What sequence of events led to the patient's death? What was found at autopsy?

Selected Reading

Faloon WW: Hepatobiliary effects of obesity and weight-reducing surgery. Semin Liver Dis 8:229–236, 1988.

Klein S, Nealon WH: Hepatobiliary abnormalities associated with total parenteral nutrition. Semin Liver Dis 8:237–246, 1988.

Lerman RH, Cave DR: Medical and surgical management of obesity. Adv Intern Med 34:127–163, 1989.

20 ADENOCARCINOMA OF THE SIGMOID COLON

Key Words | colon cancer, metastatic disease, bronchopneumonia

CASE

The patient was a 68-year-old woman who had had a left hemicolectomy five years previously for adenocarcinoma of the sigmoid colon. A metastatic lesion to the lower lobe of her right lung developed three years later, for which she was given unknown chemotherapy followed by lobectomy.[1] Computed tomography of the abdomen six months later showed multiple filling defects in the liver and left adrenal gland. During the next four months, the patient was given three courses of chemotherapy consisting of CCNU, streptozocin, and fluorouracil (5-FU).[2] The course was complicated by fever of unknown origin and chemotherapy-induced granulocytopenia and anemia. The serum carcinoembryonic antigen level two months before admission was 1,950 ng/ml (normal, <5 ng/ml). She noticed swelling of the left calf during the week preceding admission.[3]

The patient was admitted for a fourth course of chemotherapy. She had the evidence of metastatic adenocarcinoma noted above, deep vein thromboses of her left leg, and volume depletion with hyperkalemia; stool were positive by guaiac test for occult blood.[4] After she received intravenous hydration therapy, her hematocrit decreased from 31% to 25% (normal, 35 to 47%). She was transfused with 4 units of packed red blood cells. On admission, blood samples were drawn for culture

DISCUSSION

1. The sigmoid colon is the most common site of origin of adenocarcinoma of the colon. An isolated metastasis is sometimes removed surgically to reduce the tumor burden and consequently improve the chances of successful chemotherapy. Many patients either never knew or cannot remember with which drugs they were previously treated.
2. The multiple filling defects probably represent nodules of metastatic tumor. CCNU, also known as lomustine, is a nitrosurea compound that acts as an alkylating agent. Streptozocin is an antibiotic with cytotoxic activity. 5-FU is a pyrimidine analog.
3. Many chemotherapeutic agents kill rapidly dividing cells in bone marrow; this potentially leads to decreased production of leukocytes, erythrocytes, and platelets. Carcinoembryonic antigen is present in some gastrointestinal cancers. Serum carcinoembryonic antigen levels provide a useful indicator for the body's tumor burden and may indicate the presence of metastasis or recurrent carcinoma. Serum levels in early cancer are usually too low to be useful for diagnosis. Swelling of one but not the other leg suggests a local process such as venous or lymphatic obstruction rather than a systemic process such as cardiac, renal, or hepatic failure. Bedridden patients are vulnerable to venous stasis with resulting deep vein thromboses.
4. Stools testing positive for occult blood suggest that the patient was bleeding from an unknown site, pos-

125

CASE

because of fever, tachycardia, and tachypnea in the absence of localizing signs; she was treated with the antibiotics cefoxitin and gentamicin.[5] A venogram of her left leg was performed on the next day. Left deep vein thrombosis with questionable blood clot in the left common iliac vein was diagnosed. After therapy with heparin followed by warfarin, the patient's prothrombin time doubled and her partial thromboplastin time tripled.[6] She developed bilateral alveolar infiltrate with tachypnea on the third hospital day. Her continuing dyspnea was treated with oxygen supplementation.[7]

The patient's blood urea nitrogen and serum creatinine levels rose over the next few days. She also developed persistent hypotension, which was only partially reversed with pressor agents. Her serum carcinoembryonic antigen level at that time was 2,360 ng/ml. Also, she continued to have increased prothrombin and partial thromboplastin times, despite withdrawal of the anticoagulation therapy.[8] Her condition continued to deteriorate, and she remained dyspneic. A sputum culture on the ninth hospital day showed heavy growth of *Streptococcus viridans*, moderate growth of non-hemolytic streptococci, and light growth of *Pseudomonas aeruginosa*. Her antibiotic therapy was switched to pipericillin and erythromycin. Vitamin K therapy was administered to correct her coagulopathy. She remained in a dyspneic state and died 15 days after admission.[9]

At autopsy, the patient had widespread metastatic disease involving the left adrenal gland, liver, right upper and middle lobes of the lungs, peripancreatic and portahepatic lymph nodes, and right paratracheal and hilar lymph nodes (Figs. 20-1 to 20-3). There was extensive necrosis of tumor, most probably attributable to chemotherapy.[10] Bilateral acute bronchopneumonia was present. Two small pulmonary emboli involved the left upper and right middle lobes and were associated with hemorrhagic infarct. The likely source of these emboli was a left common iliac vein thrombus.[11] In summary, this patient had widespread metastatic colonic adenocarcinoma

DISCUSSION

sibly a tumor in the bowel. The reason for the patient's volume depletion was not clear, but may have been simply inadequate fluid intake coupled with increased losses due to fever.

5. It is common for rehydration of a substantially dehydrated patient to significantly lower the hematocrit. Patients with cancer are vulnerable to infection in part because normal physiological barriers are often disrupted by the tumor and in part because systemic cancer often produces a moderate degree of immunosuppression.

6. A venogram is a radiograph of a vein filled with contrast medium. Deep vein thromboses can be a source of pulmonary emboli. Heparin, but not warfarin, is given intravenously and is consequently used as an anticoagulant first.

7. The bilateral alveolar infiltrate suggests that pneumonia had involved both lungs. The patient was already vulnerable to dyspnea since one lobe had been previously removed and there was probably new metastatic tumor involving the remaining portions of the lungs.

8. Rising blood urea nitrogen and serum creatinine levels suggest that she was developing renal failure, possibly related to lowered blood pressure or metastatic tumor. Decreasing blood pressure suggests that this patient was developing symptoms of sepsis. High carcinoembryonic antigen levels indicate that the patient's tumor mass was still large, despite chemotherapy. In a seriously ill patient who is receiving anticoagulants, synthesis of clotting factors by the liver may be reduced. Such a patient will recover more slowly from anticoagulant therapy than will a healthier patient.

9. Since the results of the patient's sputum cultures were difficult to interpret, she was treated with broad-spectrum antibiotics. Therapy with vitamin K tends to increase liver synthesis of clotting factors that require the vitamin during their synthesis.

10. The liver and lungs are common metastatic sites for colon cancer since the venous drainage from the gastrointestinal tract is first through the portal system and then from the heart to the pulmonary system. The predilection of adenocarcinoma to metastasize to the adrenal glands is well known but less well under-

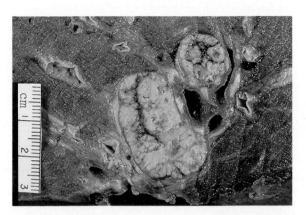

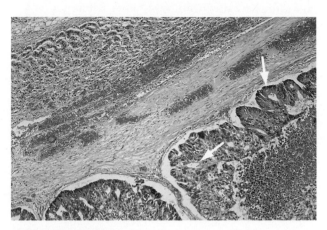

Fig. 20-1. Adenocarcinoma metastatic to the lung (gross specimen). This patient's adenocarcinoma of the colon has metastasized to form large, whitish, pulmonary nodules. The black interior of the nodules is probably due to necrosis with hemorrhage. Such necrosis commonly occurs when growth of a tumor nodule exceeds the blood supply to the tumor.

Fig. 20-2. Metastatic tumor involving the adrenal gland (low power photomicrograph, hematoxylin and eosin). Adrenal tissue in upper left, tumor in lower right. Hemorrhage is present in the fibrous tissue and in the adrenal parenchyma. The tumor forms glandlike structures *(arrows)* resembling colonic epithelium. An area of tumor necrosis with hemorrhage is present *(lower right)*.

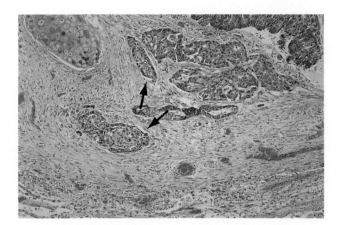

Fig. 20-3. Adenocarcinoma involving the lung (high power photomicrograph, hematoxylin and eosin). This field is taken from an area adjacent to a bronchus (note the cartilage in upper left corner). Slitlike spaces *(arrows)* can be observed at the edges of the small masses of tumor cells in the center of the field. These slitlike spaces suggest that the tumor is present in lymphatic channels and is metastasizing by a lymphatic route.

CASE

and ultimately died from respiratory failure secondary to acute bronchopneumonia and pulmonary embolism.

DISCUSSION

stood. It may be that the glands are vulnerable in part because they are highly vascularized.

11. Although anticoagulant therapy is safer for patients with deep vein thromboses than no anticoagulant therapy, it does not completely remove the risk of pulmonary embolism.

Adenocarcinoma of the Colon

Adenocarcinoma of the colon is the most common gastrointestinal cancer and usually affects patients older than 50. Many patients with colon cancer do not experience symptoms until late in the disease, when therapy is difficult. Complete obstruction of the bowel is rare. Partial obstruction may result only in a decrease in the size of the stool and altered bowel habits. Although bleeding can occur, it is often occult and may be missed if the patient is otherwise asymptomatic. The possibility of colon cancer should consequently be considered in older patients with iron deficiency anemia. Other complications include perforation leading to peritonitis, enterocutaneous and rectovaginal fistulas, and bladder symptoms due to compression or invasion by the tumor. Many colon cancers produce carcinoembryonic antigen, but unfortunately the serum levels do not become significantly elevated until the cancer is widespread. Consequently, the serum carcinoembryonic antigen level is not a useful screening test for early lesions. It is, however, used to monitor patients for recurrent disease and as a diagnostic clue in the evaluation of patients with metastases of unknown origin.

The very low incidence of adenocarcinoma of the colon in some regions of Africa has suggested that dietary factors, possibly either low fiber or high fat and animal protein content, may be risk factors for the development of colon cancer. There also appears to be an important relationship, whose details have not yet been fully elucidated, between benign polyps and later development of cancer. Adenomatous polyps tend to precede colon cancer by 10 to 15 years; dysplastic foci are often found in adenomatous polyps; and prophylactic removal of polyps can substantially reduce the risk of subsequent cancer development. All individuals over the age of 50 years are advised to undergo screening by rigid or flexible sigmoidoscopy. Such screening can detect both premalignant polyps and tumors at a sufficiently early stage that a cure may be possible.

Questions

1. Discuss the epidemiology of adenocarcinoma of the colon. How can adenocarcinoma of the colon present? What types of complications can occur?
2. Summarize the patient's clinical history. What evidence of metastatic carcinoma did she have? How was she treated? What was the rationale for each therapy? Where were tumors found at autopsy?
3. What complications of her disease or its therapy did this patient experience? Why was she vulnerable to these complications? Discuss the physical findings and laboratory studies that help to clarify the patient's clinical status with respect to these processes.

Selected Reading

Block GE: Colon cancer: diagnosis and prognosis in the elderly. Geriatrics 44:45–47, 52–53, 1989.

Carden DL, Smith JK: Pneumonias. Emerg Med Clin N Am 7:255–278, 1989.

LIVER AND PANCREAS

21 MASSIVE HEPATIC LACERATION AFTER BLUNT TRAUMA TO THE ABDOMEN

Key Words | trauma, hepatic laceration, hemorrhage

CASE

A 31-year-old man sustained blunt trauma to the abdomen in an automobile accident. After lying at the edge of the road for approximately 20 minutes, he was brought to the emergency room of a community hospital, where he was found to be hypotensive. Resuscitative measures including transfusion of fluids were administered.[1] Exploratory laparotomy revealed a massive stellate laceration through the central portion of the liver. There was extensive intra-abdominal hemorrhage, arising mostly from the central portion of the porta hepatis. The right hepatic vein was transected, as well as several of its tributaries.[2] The gallbladder was involved, and a cholecystectomy was performed. The common bile duct was explored and reconstructed over a T-tube.[3] The arterial supply to the right lobe of the liver was preserved. Additional intrahepatic damage was demonstrated by intraoperative cholangiograms.[4]

After surgery, the patient was sent to an intensive care unit, where he was found to have some biliary drainage from the T-tube, but also extensive biliary drainage from Penrose drains inserted into the peritoneal cavity. He was then transferred to a university hospital. Three days after the accident, a right trisegmentectomy was performed

DISCUSSION

1. The patient's hypotension suggested that serious blood loss may have occurred. Transfusion of fluids was used to restore volume and limit the risks of shock.

2. Information about a patient's condition can be obtained more rapidly and safely by laparotomy than by conventional exploratory surgery. The phrase *stellate* is used when a laceration is composed of multiple tears centered on a small region. The liver is susceptible to stellate lacerations because it is a large, relatively mobile organ that is tethered in a small area by the porta hepatis. Such lacerations commonly tear at least some of the vessels in the porta hepatis and can produce massive hemorrhage. Surgical reconstruction involves principally debridement of damaged tissue and repair of as many damaged vessels and ducts as possible.

3. When the bile duct system is so damaged that simple suturing of any tears is not feasible, artificial tubing is used in reconstruction. The T shape of the prosthesis permits the pancreatic and bile ducts to be joined, approximating the normal duct configuration. Reconstruction of the gallbladder is usually not attempted since the organ is not necessary for adequate gastrointestinal function and is easier to remove than repair.

4. Ideally, the liver parenchyma requires perfusion by

131

CASE

(Fig. 21-1). During this surgery, the biliary system was reconstructed by left hepatojejunostomy.[5] Postoperatively, the patient appeared to be stable. On the morning following surgery, he experienced a sudden cardiorespiratory arrest from which he could not be resuscitated. The history was significant in that he had been noted to have cardiac arrhythmias when he was younger.[6]

At autopsy, a large proportion of the patient's remaining liver was found to be viable and showed changes associated with active regeneration (Fig. 21-2). Prominent cholestasis was present. This was considered to probably be a feature of regeneration rather than an indication of a problem with biliary drainage, which appeared to be adequate. Some areas of the liver did show centrilobular necrosis, indicating inadequate blood supply. Substantially more than half of the remaining liver showed no evidence of ischemic damage.[7]

There was evidence of prominent embolization of fat droplets into the systemic and pulmonary circulations, which apparently resulted in substantial vascular engorgement in the kidneys and lung (Fig. 21-3). Such embolization may peak several days after trauma, and this process may have contributed to the patient's death. Additionally, the patient had a history of arrhythmias and autopsy evidence of left ventricular hypertrophy. Local obstruction of cardiac vessels by lipid emboli might have precipitated an arrhythmia with resulting cardiorespiratory arrest.[8]

DISCUSSION

both portal vein and hepatic artery systems. The degree of preservation of the blood supply is a major determinant in the decision whether to remove or preserve portions of the liver. Cholangiograms are radiographs of the liver and surrounding area taken after injection of a contrast medium that is excreted into the biliary system.

5. Penrose drains are placed through the abdominal wall to drain the peritoneal cavity by gravity drainage. They permit monitoring of peritoneal fluids and diminish the risk of serious peritonitis. A right trisegmentectomy consists of removing the large right lobe of the liver plus the medial segment containing the porta hepatis. This procedure badly disrupts biliary drainage. Connecting the remaining large intrahepatic bile ducts in the small left lobe to the intestine by a hepatojejunostomy is a method of reconstructing the biliary tree. This extensive surgery is feasible because of the remarkable regenerative ability of the liver. Most of the volume of the original liver can be restored, via hypertrophy of the remaining lobe, in typically less than two months. Regeneration can also occur in many other liver diseases. It is most effective if the original insult no longer remains to damage the regenerating liver and if the underlying connective tissue structure of the liver remains intact.

6. There are only a relatively few common reasons for sudden death after surgery; arrhythmias, pulmonary emboli, and massive hemorrhage are the most significant.

7. The speed with which the liver can regenerate is indicated by the fact that the patient's liver, four days after the accident and only one day after surgery, already showed widespread evidence of regeneration. Cholestasis can occur in a regenerating liver because development of a working biliary system may lag behind development of functioning hepatocytes. The central region of a classical lobule, near the branches of the central hepatic vein, is the region most vulnerable to ischemia. Cells in that area experience the lowest oxygen tension as they are furthest from both the hepatic artery and the vein emanating from the portal triad.

8. The lipid present in the membranes of a cell's organelles and plasmalemma becomes available for phagocytosis if the cell dies. However, if a large volume of soft tissue (e.g., liver) suddenly dies, the body's ca-

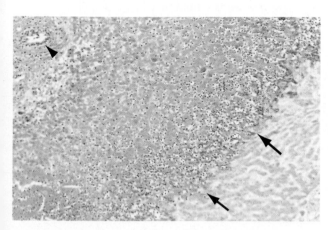

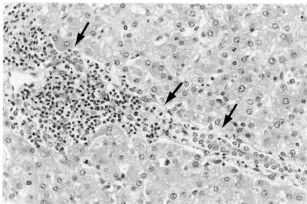

Fig. 21-1. Necrotic liver (low power photomicrograph, hematoxylin and eosin). This necrotic liver was removed during the patient's abdominal surgery following his automobile accident. Viable tissue is present at the upper left; coagulation necrosis is present at the lower right. A relatively healthy bile duct is present in the upper left corner *(arrowhead)*. Most of the hepatocytes in the field are dead, as indicated by the absence of hepatocyte nuclei. A prominent neutrophilic infiltrate *(arrows)* marks the boundary between coagulated necrotic hepatocytes and liquefied tissue.

Fig. 21-2. Regenerating liver (high power photomicrograph, hematoxylin and eosin). This liver sample was taken at autopsy. Despite the massive death of cells illustrated in the previous figure, the patient's liver had markedly regenerated. A bile duct *(arrows)* courses diagonally through the field and is partially surrounded by a lymphocytic infiltrate. In contrast, the hepatic parenchyma appears healthy. Double nuclei are present in many hepatocytes and indicate that active regeneration is occurring.

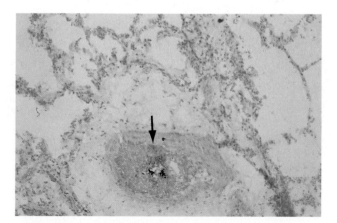

Fig. 21-3. Fat emboli in the lung (high power photomicrograph, oil red O). The arteriole at the bottom center contains lipid that stains reddish with oil red O *(arrow)*. This patient's lipid emboli were present in many tissues and were probably derived from lipid in the massive amount of necrotic membranes present in the dead liver.

DISCUSSION

pacity to process the lipid may be exceeded. Lipid droplets may enter the circulation and lodge in smaller-diameter arteries and arterioles. Such lipid droplets behave like other emboli and are capable of impairing perfusion to tissues and causing congestion in vessels proximal to the obstruction. Lipid emboli also arise from trauma to fat or fractures of long bones with resultant fat or bone marrow emboli.

Chest and Abdominal Trauma

Trauma to the chest may, by a variety of mechanisms, impair the ability to breathe. Rib fracture is common. A broken rib that is forced into the underlying lung may cause laceration, hemothorax, and pneumothorax. Multiple ribs can be fractured in several locations, as may happen in blunt trauma against an automobile steering wheel. When this happens, a flail chest may be produced in which the damaged portion of the rib cage paradoxically moves in during inspiration and out during expiration. Pulmonary contusion can cause alveolar rupture with hemorrhage and transudation of fluid. The resulting obstruction of airways and bronchi can produce atelectasis of distal alveoli. This process can be exacerbated if the patient has been treated excessively with fluid replacement in an attempt to maintain blood pressure. The trachea and bronchi can be crushed between the sternum and vertebrae during rapid deceleration in an automobile accident. Such injuries can produce either occlusion of the airways or massive air leaks that prevent the lungs from expanding during inspiration. Blunt injury to the heart can occur by the same mechanism. Rupture of a cardiac chamber occurs in some immediately fatal injuries. Penetrating injuries of the heart or major vessels can lead to rapid exsanguination. Penetrating injuries to the diaphragm may impair breathing and may also predispose to later herniation of abdominal contents into the thoracic cavity.

The principal risks of abdominal trauma are hemorrhage, rupture of organs, and blunt trauma to solid organs. Hemorrhage can result from injury to large vessels or serious liver injury. The biliary tree is also very vulnerable to injury and must be surgically reconstructed if damaged. Solid organs, such as the spleen, pancreas, and liver, can rupture during blunt trauma.

Surgical debridement and possibly removal of the involved organ may be necessary. A perforated gastrointestinal tract should be repaired or badly damaged portions resected. Aggressive antibiotic therapy may be required to control peritonitis, which, in this setting, commonly involves multiple organisms. Urine leakage can occur after injury to the bladder or ureters. Blunt trauma to the kidney may require partial or total nephrectomy. Surgical exploration is performed if fever, hypotension, or localizing signs are present and often if there are injuries commonly associated with abdominal organ trauma, such as rib, spine, or pelvic fractures.

Questions

1. Why was this man brought to the emergency room? Discuss the types of injury that can occur after blunt trauma to the abdomen. What injury did this patient experience? How was the injury diagnosed?
2. What surgical repair was initially performed? Why was the patient transferred to a university hospital? Why did he have a second hepatic surgery? Was the surgery technically successful?
3. What happened postoperatively? What cardiac problem had the patient had when younger? Describe the patient's liver at autopsy. What other organs were seriously affected by the liver injury?

Selected Reading

Langdale L, Schecter WP: Critical care complications in the trauma patient. Crit Care Clin 2:839–852, 1986.

Sheldon GF, Rutledge R: Hepatic trauma. Adv Surg 22:179–193, 1989.

Smedira N, Schecter WP: Blunt abdominal trauma. Emerg Med Clin N Am 7:631–645, 1989.

22 BUDD-CHIARI SYNDROME COMPLICATING POLYCYTHEMIA VERA

Key Words | polycythemia, intravascular coagulation, Budd-Chiari syndrome

CASE

A 57-year-old woman was admitted after experiencing malaise, nausea, and vomiting for two and one-half weeks. Abdominal pain developed shortly before admission. Liver function tests showed elevations in serum aspartate aminotransferase (SGOT) to 1,078 U/ml (normal, <37 U/ml), serum alanine aminotransferase (SGPT) to 1,430 U/ml (normal, <34 U/ml), and serum bilirubin to 2.4 mg/100 ml (normal, 0.3 to 1.5 mg/100 ml). The hematocrit was 66.8% (normal, 35 to 47%).[1] An abdominal ultrasonogram showed ascitic fluid, an enlarged spleen, and an enlarged liver. Peritoneal fluid was tapped, revealing a transudate with no malignant cells and no bacteria on culture. Hepatitis B surface antigen was absent; the serum amylase level was normal. The α-fetoprotein level was also normal, and results of tests for anti-mitochondrial and anti-smooth muscle antibodies were negative.[2] Occlusion of the hepatic veins was demonstrated by an inferior vena cavagram, and a diagnosis of Budd-Chiari syndrome was made. Results of hematological studies indicated hypercellular bone marrow with erythroid hyperplasia and depleted iron stores; the patient was considered to have polycythemia vera.[3]

DISCUSSION

1. Malaise, nausea, vomiting, and abdominal pain are nonspecific symptoms that suggest abdominal disease. Aspartate aminotransferase (also called glutamic-oxaloacetic transaminase) and alanine aminotransferase (also called glutamic-pyruvic transaminase) are enzymes that interconvert tricarboxylic acid cycle intermediates and amino acids. Elevation of these liver function enzymes suggests hepatocellular damage. The elevated hematocrit suggests that either a relative or absolute polycythemia was present. The clinical picture was unclear, and a number of screening tests were ordered to exclude a variety of diagnostic possibilities.

2. Ascites, enlarged spleen, and enlarged liver are again relatively nonspecific findings. The presence of malignant cells or bacteria in the ascites fluid would have suggested, respectively, disseminated cancer and peritonitis. Chronic active hepatitis due to hepatitis B virus infection was excluded by the lack of surface antigen. The normal serum amylase suggests that pancreatic disease was not part of the patient's problem. α-Fetoprotein is a fetal enzyme that is expressed by some cancers; high α-fetoprotein levels, if present, would suggest hepatocellular cancer. The negative results for anti-mitochondrial and anti-

CASE

The patient's epigastric pain, nausea, and vomiting persisted. She became more lethargic and had an episode of hematochezia and melena. A nasogastric aspirate contained no blood, and sigmoidoscopy showed no lesions.[4] Her prothrombin and partial thromboplastin times both rose to approximately twice control values. The serum aspartate aminotransferase and alanine aminotransferase decreased, respectively to 445 and 565 U/ml; bilirubin rose to 4.5 mg/100 ml. The platelet count decreased from high normal to low normal. The white blood cell count rose from 19,500/mm^3 to 44,700/mm^3 (normal, 4,500 to 11,000/mm^3).[5]

The initial treatment plan included intravenous hydration, nutritional support, and lactulose. One week after admission, the patient developed fever, and fluid with a white blood cell count of 10,800/mm^3 and erythrocyte count of 126,000/mm^3 was recovered by paracentesis. Gram-positive cocci were reportedly seen when paracentesis fluid was stained. These findings were consistent with bacterial peritonitis, thought to be possibly spontaneous bacterial peritonitis. Antibiotic therapy with ampicillin and tobramycin was begun. Later, clindamycin was added.[6] During the patient's hospital course, her blood urea nitrogen and serum creatinine levels rose to 35 mg/100 ml (normal, 6 to 20 mg/100 ml) and 2.3 mg/100 ml (normal, 0.5 to 1.4 mg/100 ml), respectively. Her hematocrit fell to 32.3%. She was given multiple transfusions of fresh-frozen plasma and packed red blood cells. Her condition worsened, and she became unresponsive. She followed a progressively worsening course and died ten days after admission. At the family's request, no resuscitative efforts were instituted. Results of cultures from blood and peritoneal fluid specimens obtained two days before death showed no growth.[7]

Autopsy revealed organized thrombi occluding the hepatic veins, inferior vena cava, portal veins, splenic vein, and superior mesenteric vein (Fig. 22-1). The liver showed severe centrilobular congestion with complete atrophy of centrilobular liver cells and hemorrhage into the Disse space with adjacent empty sinusoids.[8] Many portal vein

DISCUSSION

smooth muscle antibodies tend to exclude a chronic autoimmune process involving the liver.

3. Occlusion of the hepatic veins produces the Budd-Chiari syndrome. The clinical presentation may follow either an acute or chronic course. In the acute form, the clinical presentation includes abdominal pain, rapid enlargement of the liver, and massive ascites; death may occur within hours to approximately one month. The chronic form follows an insidious course with milder symptoms, which may lead to death only after months or years. Erythroid hyperplasia suggests that the patient's polycythemia was absolute, rather than a relative polycythemia due to fluid loss; polycythemia vera, rather than secondary polycythemia, is suggested by the absence of respiratory symptoms or any other identifiable case of increased hematopoiesis. Chronic erythropoiesis often consumes bone marrow iron stores. Occlusion of the hepatic veins was probably due to clotting of hyperviscous blood, which was prone to stasis and was a consequence of the patient's polycythemia. The patient's abdominal pain, nausea, and vomiting may have been due to ischemia of abdominal organs.

4. The patient's lethargy was of serious concern because it suggests that she may have been experiencing severe liver failure and that a toxic metabolic state may have been developing. *Hematochezia* refers to the passage of grossly bloody stools; *melena* refers to the passage of tarry stools containing altered blood. The absence of blood in the nasogastric aspirate suggests that the bleeding was below the level of the duodenum. Since no lesions were visible by sigmoidoscopy, the bleeding appeared to be from above the sigmoid colon.

5. The patient's rising prothrombin and partial thromboplastin times suggest that she was developing a coagulopathy secondary to decreased synthesis of clotting factors by her dying liver. Since aspartate aminotransferase and alanine aminotransferase are released by damaged hepatocytes, falling levels of these enzymes are usually good prognostic signs since they indicate resolving of acute hepatocellular disease. However, in this case, the falling serum enzyme levels may have reflected death of so much of the patient's liver that large numbers of hepatocytes are no longer able to leak enzyme. The decrease in platelet counts probably reflects their consumption by the patient's

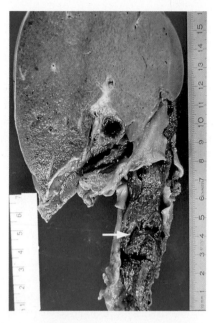

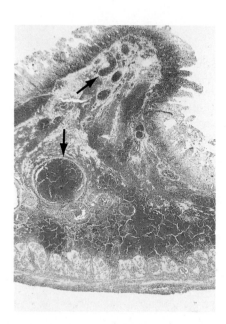

Fig. 22-1. Thrombosis involving the inferior vena cava (gross photograph). The liver is above, and the vena cava is below. A massive thrombus is present in the inferior vena cava *(arrow)*. Similar thrombi were present throughout the portal venous system.

Fig. 22-2. Infarcted small bowel (low power photomicrograph, hematoxylin and eosin). This area of infarcted bowel shows massive hemorrhage in the submucosa. Several veins containing clotted blood are apparent *(arrows)*; these clots were probably contiguous with the clots in the portal system and liver. Since the blockage to blood flow was in the venous system, arterial pressures were maintained and caused rupture of arterioles and capillaries, with subsequent hemorrhage, as the tissue died of hypoxia.

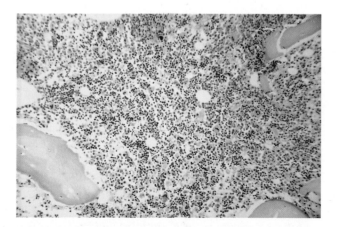

Fig. 22-3. Hypercellular bone marrow (low power photomicrograph, hematoxylin and eosin). The marrow is markedly hypercellular, with almost complete replacement of the normal marrow fat cells by predominatly erythrocyte precursors. In polycythemia vera, although erythrocyte precursors predominate, granulocytes and megakaryocytes also can be present in increased numbers.

CASE

branches contained recent occlusive thrombi. The small bowel was extensively infarcted (Fig. 22-2). Pneumatosis cystoides intestinalis of the colon was present. Examination of the bone marrow revealed hypercellularity with erythroid hyperplasia and absent iron stores, consistent with polycythemia vera; extramedullary hematopoiesis was present in the spleen (Fig. 22-3). The cause of death was considered to be liver failure and small bowel infarction with gastrointestinal hemorrhage in a patient with polycythemia vera, extensive venous thrombosis, and Budd-Chiari syndrome.[9]

DISCUSSION

clotting blood. Rising leukocyte counts suggest that she may have been developing a serious infection.

6. Lactulose is useful in the treatment of hepatic encephalopathy because it causes a mild diarrhea and its metabolites can bind ammonia. Some physicians might have treated this patient with anticoagulants on the theory that judicious use of anticoagulants might prevent the formation of clots due to stasis while actually reducing hemorrhaging by tending to restore serum levels of clotting factors. The presence of bacteria in the ascitic fluid suggests that the patient had developed peritonitis. Bowel ischemia due to poor venous drainage through the portal system may have been a predisposing factor. Since no specific organism had been identified and a bowel source, with potentially multiple organisms, was suspected, broad-spectrum antibiotics were used that had activity against gram-positive, gram-negative, and anaerobic organisms.

7. Rising blood urea nitrogen and serum creatinine levels suggest that this patient was also developing renal failure. Her dropping hematocrit suggests that she was bleeding substantially, possibly either into the gastrointestinal tract or into the peritoneal cavity. The absence of bacteria in blood and peritoneal fluid suggests that her peritonitis had been controlled with antibiotics, but such control was obviously not adequate to prevent her death.

8. Autopsy results confirmed the polycythemia and were striking for the very widespread presence of clots in the portal and vena caval systems. These clots caused liver failure and infarction of the bowel with gastrointestinal hemorrhage. The hepatic changes associated with centrilobular congestion occur when flow through the hepatic veins is chronically impeded, either (as in this case) by probable partial occlusion of the hepatic veins over time or by a process such as congestive heart failure that produces chronic elevation of the systemic venous pressure. These changes characteristically involve death of the centrilobular hepatocytes, near the central venous system, with the portal systems often selectively preserved.

9. Infarction of the bowel occurs because venous drainage from the gastrointestinal tract into the portal system is impeded by organized thrombi throughout the superior mesenteric and portal system; hemorrhagic infarcts are characteristically produced in this setting since arterial pressures remain high and can rupture

DISCUSSION

vessels damaged by hypoxia. In pneumatosis cystoides intestinalis, numerous pockets of gas, probably formed by bacteria, are found in the wall of the gut; in this case they were related to ischemia. When extreme degrees of erythroid hyperplasia are present, for whatever reason, it is not uncommon for some erythropoiesis to occur in extramedullary sites such as the spleen, liver, or even lungs. Once Budd-Chiari syndrome is well established, the organ damage is very difficult to treat. In this patient, the outcome might have been more favorable if her polycythemia could have been diagnosed and treated before widespread thrombosis began.

Polycythemia Vera

Polycythemia vera is an idiopathic disease characterized by marked proliferation of erythrocytes. The bone marrow typically shows markedly increased hypercellularity with corresponding loss of adipose tissue. Although increased erythropoiesis is most prominent, all cell lines are often stimulated. Results of blood studies may reflect this stimulation by showing increases in the numbers of erythrocytes, leukocytes, and platelets. Bone marrow iron stores are typically reduced or nonexistent owing to the continuous consumption of iron during erythropoiesis. There is some experimental evidence that polycythemia vera may actually be similar to some chronic leukemias.

The hypercellularity present in the blood produces increased viscosity. This increased viscosity has a number of physiological effects. In the low-pressure venous system, the blood is sluggish and prone to stasis. The hepatic veins are particularly vulnerable since there has been a pressure drop across two capillary beds, rather than just one. Consequently, a known complication of polycythemia vera is the Budd-Chiari syndrome, in which occlusion of the hepatic veins leads to hepatic congestion, necrosis, and portal hypertension. Stasis in the portal system may occur secondary to stasis in the hepatic veins, as happened in this patient. When it does, widespread infarction of the bowel and clotting of the portal system can occur. Such infarctions tend to be associated with hemorrhage because the arterial system

is still patent, and blood tends to be forced out of the arteries and capillary beds into the necrotic adjacent tissue. The infarctions are also associated with loss of function of the involved organs and risk of peritonitis if perforation occurs.

Questions

1. How did this patient present? Which of her initial studies gave abnormal results? What diseases should have been considered in the differential diagnosis of her problems? How was the diagnosis finally made?
2. What is Budd-Chiari syndrome? What is polycythemia vera? How were these conditions related in this patient? Explain how they account for her clinical findings.
3. Discuss the patient's hospital course. What additional complications did she experience? How were these related to her polycythemia vera? How was she treated? What was found at autopsy?

Selected Reading

Hocking WG, Golde DW: Polycythemia: evaluation and management. Blood Rev 3:59–65, 1989.

Patterson WP, Caldwell CW, Doll DC: Hyperviscosity syndromes and coagulopathies. Semin Oncol 17:210–216, 1990.

Stanley P: Budd-Chiari syndrome. Radiology 170:625–627, 1989.

23 OBSTRUCTIVE CHOLESTASIS AND PERFORATED VISCUS IN A PATIENT WITH END-STAGE RENAL DISEASE

Key Words | cholestasis, peritonitis, chronic renal failure

CASE

A 70-year-old woman had a long history of end-stage renal disease thought to be secondary to glomerulonephritis. She had been on hemodialysis for the previous seven years.[1] She was noted to have a normocytic, normochromic anemia with normal iron stores. Over the next four months, the anemia progressed to the point that the patient's hematocrit decreased to 19% (normal, 35 to 47%). Her stools tested positive by the guaiac test for occult blood.[2] Over that period, persistent slightly high liver enzyme levels, with alanine aminotransferase (SGPT) of 60 to 100 U/ml (normal, <37 U/ml) and aspartate aminotransferase (SGOT) of 70 to 150 U/ml (normal, <34 U/ml), also developed. Results of serum bilirubin studies were initially normal and rose to a peak of 10.6 mg/100 ml of total bilirubin (normal, 0.3 to 1.5 mg/100 ml) with direct bilirubin levels of 8.9 mg/ 100 ml (normal, 0.1 to 0.4 mg/100 ml). The prothrombin and partial thromboplastin times rose to approximately twice the normal times, but

DISCUSSION

1. New problems in a patient with a chronic disease may be complications of the preexisting disease or may be due to unrelated problems.
2. Patients on chronic hemodialysis do not secrete adequate quantities of erythropoietin from their dysfunctional kidneys. The anemia produced is usually mild, but can become severe if coexisting hemorrhage is present. Stools testing positive for occult blood by the guaiac test suggest gastrointestinal bleeding, possibly due to ulcers, esophageal varices, or tumor.
3. Slightly high liver enzyme levels indicate modest hepatocellular damage. Rising bilirubin levels with conjugated (direct) bilirubin levels greater than unconjugated levels suggest obstructive jaundice, possibly due to extrahepatic causes. The prothrombin time evaluates the efficiency of the extrinsic clotting system; the partial thromboplastin time evaluates the efficiency of the intrinsic clotting system. Increased prothrombin and partial thromboplastin times suggest inadequate synthesis of serum clotting factors by the liver. Vitamin K improves the synthesis of these

141

CASE

corrected after vitamin K therapy.[3] The patient was transfused, but her hematocrit remained low and her stools remained positive for occult blood. Ultrasonograms of the pancreas and biliary tree were unremarkable. Computed tomograms of the liver and pancreas were normal. The impression at admission was that the patient's jaundice was secondary to an obstructive process, but non-A, non-B hepatitis could not be ruled out.[4]

After transfer to the university hospital, the patient began to experience multiple seizures that were only poorly controlled by antiepileptic medication. These seizures were described as focal clonic movements of her left eye, mouth, and left arm. The patient became unresponsive to voice and responded only to pain. Two computed tomograms of the head were normal. A lumbar puncture performed five days after admission showed only small quantities of erythrocytes and neutrophils.[5] A urinary tract infection with *Escherichia coli* was present and was treated with ampicillin. Although the patient had continuing jaundice and results of liver function tests were abnormal, this appeared to be a resolving process. Stools continued to test positive for occult blood, and anemia and lower gastrointestinal bleeding also continued. The patient was considered to be unable to tolerate extensive evaluation at that time. The neurological problems also persisted.[6] At 15 days after admission, she became hypotensive and acidotic and began to appear septic. Abdominal radiographs revealed the possibility of free air under the left hemidiaphragm. It was decided to give the patient comfort measures only, and she died on the 20th hospital day.[7]

At autopsy, the kidneys were noted to be very small. The atrophic cortex contained multiple cysts. Some tubules contained bile-stained material (Fig. 23-1). The collecting system had no obstructive changes.[8] The serosal surfaces of the small intestine and colon were focally covered with a purulent green material that microscopically revealed a fulminant acute peritonitis.[9] The patient's progressive jaundice appeared to be due to extrahepatic obstruction since both the common bile and pancreatic ducts were dilated and contained intraluminal concretions. The liver showed portal fibrosis, cholangiolar duct prolifer-

DISCUSSION

factors. Such therapy can consequently restore prothrombin and partial thromboplastin times to normal in some patients.

4. The persistent low hematocrit after transfusion suggests that the patient was continuing to hemorrhage substantially. Although the results of her bilirubin studies were consistent with extrahepatic biliary obstruction, it proved difficult to identify the reason for this obstruction by computed tomography and ultrasonography.

5. Patients with hepatic failure can experience neurological symptoms as a result of their disturbed metabolic state. Seizures occur relatively early, whereas coma occurs later if hepatic failure continues to progress. Seizures due to a disordered metabolism are not always easily controlled with antiepileptic medication. Although hepatic failure and other metabolic disturbances are possible explanations of this patient's developing coma, other causes should also be evaluated. Neither computed tomography nor lumbar puncture provided definitive information, but they did tend to exclude tumor, meningitis, and cranial hemorrhage.

6. It is not always appropriate to subject a seriously ill patient to extensive evaluation since many diagnostic procedures are invasive, require considerable cooperation from the patient, and may push a metabolically unstable patient into a crisis. The longer that neurological symptoms persist in a patient with hepatic dysfunction, the greater the chance that permanent neurological deficits, including coma, will be produced.

7. Bacterial sepsis causes both metabolic acidosis and hypotension. Diagnostic possibilities for infection in this patient that should be considered include urinary tract infection, aspiration or other pneumonia, bedsores, and abdominal infection possibly related to the hepatic dysfunction. Free air under the diaphragm indicates that perforation of the gastrointestinal tract, most probably the bowel, has occurred. It further suggests that peritonitis is the cause of sepsis in this patient. The decision to give comfort measures only was probably based on both the patient's poor neurological state and her unstable physiological condition, which would not have permitted surgery. Antibiotic treatment without surgery is often unsuccessful because the presumed perforation of a hollow viscus provides a continuing source of antibiotic-resistant organisms.

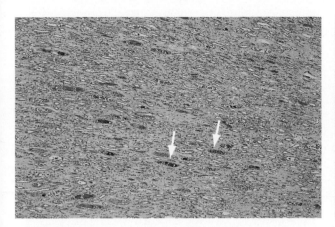

Fig. 23-1. Bile casts in the renal medulla (low power photomicrograph, hematoxylin and eosin). Bile-stained material *(arrows)* fills multiple tubules in the renal medulla. Such material is usually observed only when serum bilirubin levels are high and significant excretion of conjugated bilirubin is occurring by renal, rather than hepatic, routes.

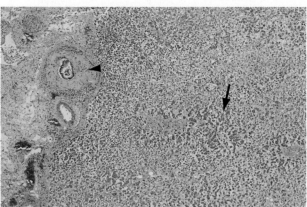

Fig. 23-2. Hepatic bile stasis (low power photomicrograph, hematoxylin and eosin). Obstruction of the biliary drainage of the liver has led to a decrease in size, and in some cases to the death, of many hepatocytes. In a few areas *(arrow)*, the hepatocytes are relatively well preserved. In the upper left, the tissue of the liver hilum is present. A thick rim of fibrous tissue can be seen surrounding part of an extrahepatic bile duct *(arrowhead)*.

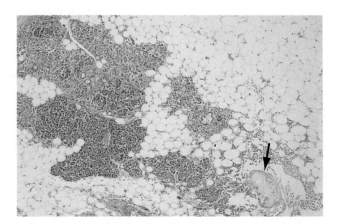

Fig. 23-3. Pancreatic fibrosis (low power photomicrograph, hematoxylin and eosin). Relatively normal pancreatic ancini stain darkly *(lower left)*. In the upper left, many acini have been replaced by fibrosis. In the lower right, necrotic fat with calcification *(arrow)* is present.

CASE

ation, and bile stasis (Fig. 23-2). The pancreas showed interstitial fibrosis (Fig. 23-3).[10] Although this hepatobiliary disease was certainly debilitating, the hypotension and sepsis were the conditions that directly led to the patient's death. *Enterobacter cloacae* was found in cultures of spleen and lung specimens. Staphylococci and *Candida stellatoidea* were also found. Supporting evidence of sepsis and hypotension included segmental ischemic colitis, polymorphonuclear leukocyte infiltrate in the spleen, multiple adrenal microinfarcts, and hypotensive hepatic changes. Marked peripancreatic fat necrosis with mild acute pancreatitis was also present. An exact point of perforation in the gastrointestinal tract was not identified but was presumably within the segment of friable ischemic colon.[11] Examination of the brain and spinal cord was not performed at the request of the family. The cause of death was considered to be sepsis in a patient with obstructive cholestasis and end-stage renal disease.

DISCUSSION

8. Small kidneys with atrophic cortex are typical of end-stage kidneys in which damage, from whatever original cause, has caused extensive loss of tissue with replacement by fibrosis. Renal cysts are a common incidental finding at autopsy.

9. The purulent green material is pus, and its presence proves the peritonitis suspected clinically. In fulminant acute peritonitis, accumulations of neutrophils, necrotic material, and sometimes focal hemorrhage dominate the microscopic picture.

10. The intraluminal concretions are bile stones. Even though extrahepatic obstruction could not be documented before the patient's death, the autopsy results did confirm its presence. The presence of stones suggests that the patient's hepatic disease was probably unrelated to her renal disease. Bile duct proliferation can occur either idiopathically or in the setting of bile obstruction, perhaps as a response to increased intraluminal pressures. Portal fibrosis is a relatively nonspecific finding, suggesting replacement of hepatocytes adjacent to the portal triad by fibrosis.

11. *Enterobacter cloacae* is a gastrointestinal organism; the other organisms noted were probably acquired from the oropharynx. Sepsis can produce both hypotension and disseminated intravascular coagulation, and consequently changes due to ischemia or infarction in multiple organs are characteristically observed at autopsy. Segmental ischemic colitis probably reflects the presence of thrombi in some mesenteric vessels. Since both coagulation and thrombolytic pathways are activated in disseminated intravascular coagulation, the thrombi that caused infarction may have dissolved by the time of autopsy. The adrenal glands, with their high metabolic requirements, are particularly vulnerable to shock-induced damage. Peripancreatic fat necrosis can be produced by occlusion of the pancreatic duct or by ischemic damage to the pancreas. In this case, since only mild acute pancreatitis was present, ischemic damage related to the patient's sepsis appears more probable than pancreatic duct occlusion, even though the presence of intraluminal concretions in the bile duct also raises the possibility of occlusion. A specific site of perforation or of hemorrhage in a bowel is not always identified at autopsy since such lesions may be small.

Hyperbilirubinemia

Jaundice is present in patients with elevated bilirubin levels. Bilirubin is a degradation product of the heme moiety of hemoglobin and is formed by reticuloendothelial cells in the bone marrow, liver, and spleen. Hepatocytes remove bilirubin from serum by conjugating it with glucuronic acid and then excreting the conjugated bilirubin into the biliary system and thence into the stool. Excessive production of bilirubin or interruption of the processes leading to its secretion can lead to hyperbilirubinemia and jaundice. In an adult without known inherited metabolic deficits, high levels of unconjugated bilirubin in the absence of both high levels of conjugated bilirubin and elevations in liver enzymes suggest excessive bilirubin production, possibly due to hemolysis or ineffective erythropoiesis. The causes of conjugated hyperbilirubinemia are more diverse and reflect the variety of ways in which cholestasis can occur. Extrahepatic obstruction can occur in the biliary tree as a result of gallstones, strictures, cysts, diverticula, or carcinoma. Pancreatic disease, including carcinoma, pseudocysts, or chronic pancreatitis, can also produce extrahepatic obstruction. Intrahepatic cholestasis may be caused by damage to hepatocytes from processes such as drugs, sepsis, pregnancy, or hepatitis; it may also be caused by obstruction of intrahepatic biliary tracts by diseases such as sarcoidosis, primary biliary cirrhosis, or sclerosing cholangitis.

Questions

1. Discuss this patient's medical problems. Which organ systems were involved? How did these disease processes interact?
2. What processes can cause jaundice with elevated bilirubin levels? How can these processes be distinguished? What did this patient's laboratory studies show? How were the studies interpreted?
3. What processes led to the patient's death? What was found at autopsy? How do these findings relate to the patient's clinical course?

Selected Reading

Celifarco A, Burakoff R: Noninfectious jaundice. Figuring out what's going on. Postgrad Med 84:191–193, 196–203, 1988.

Farmer PM, Mulakkan T: The pathogenesis of hepatic encephalopathy. Ann Clin Lab Sci 20:91–97, 1990.

Hallack A: Spontaneous bacterial peritonitis. Am J Gastroenterol 84:345–350, 1989.

24 END-STAGE LIVER DISEASE AND BLEEDING ESOPHAGEAL VARICES IN A PATIENT WITH CHRONIC ACTIVE HEPATITIS

Key Words | chronic active hepatitis, esophageal varices, gastrointestinal hemorrhage

CASE

A 35-year-old woman was admitted to a university hospital for evaluation for a liver transplant. Approximately 15 years previously, she became infected with hepatitis B from contaminated needles used during intravenous drug abuse.[1] The infection resolved, and the patient was asymptomatic for many years. Two years before admission, when she was still asymptomatic, a routine examination revealed elevations in liver enzymes. Six months before admission, the patient experienced progressive abdominal bloating and pedal edema. Several months later, the bloating and edema had not resolved and so the patient's liver disease was more extensively evaluated.[2] Liver function tests gave abnormal results, with aspartate aminotransferase (SGOT) of 154 U/ml (normal, <34 U/ml) and bilirubin of 2.8 mg/100 ml (normal, 0.3 to 1.5 mg/100 ml). The patient's serum was negative for hepatitis B surface antigen and positive for hepati-

DISCUSSION

1. Hepatitis B infections are typically acquired from contact with contaminated blood. Many intravenous drug abusers will pump blood in and out of the syringe to "clean" it; this increases the risk of contamination if needles and syringes are shared.

2. Carrier states, with or without chronic active disease, can develop following hepatitis B, but not hepatitis A, infection. The patient's hepatic, cardiovascular, and renal systems should all be evaluated as possible contributors to the ascites and peripheral edema. Most probably, the major contributing factors were portal hypertension secondary to hepatic cirrhosis and decreased serum albumin levels secondary to inadequate hepatic synthesis.

3. High aspartate aminotransferase levels suggest that liver cells are dying. Although hyperbilirubinemia can have diverse causes, the rising levels in this patient are probably due to intrahepatic obstruction of the biliary tree secondary to significant hepatic cir-

147

CASE

tis B core antigen. The serum also contained immunoglobulin to hepatitis B surface antigen.[3] Two months before admission to the university hospital, the patient had an episode of left lower lobe pneumonia. During this illness, her serum bilirubin level rose to 5.9 mg/100 ml. Endoscopy revealed esophageal varices. She was treated with prednisone followed by lactulose and neomycin, but her condition continued to deteriorate and she experienced increasing ascites. Her bilirubin was 11.5 mg/100 ml by one week before admission to the university hospital.[4]

The patient was transferred to the university hospital with a diagnosis of chronic active hepatitis secondary to hepatitis B infection. She was admitted for evaluation for liver transplantation. She was lethargic. Her blood pressure was 140/70 mmHg (normal, 100 to 140/60 to 90 mmHg), and her heart rate was 100/min (normal, 60 to 100/min). She was noted to have positive scleral icterus and ascites.[5] Her stools and hemorrhoids tested positive for occult blood. Laboratory data included a prothrombin time of 25.1 seconds (normal, 10.5 to 13.5 seconds), a partial thromboplastin time of 43 seconds (normal, 18 to 30 seconds), and bilirubin of 25.8 mg/100 ml. Abdominal ultrasonography showed ascites, a small liver secondary to cirrhosis, and splenomegaly[6] (Fig. 24-1).

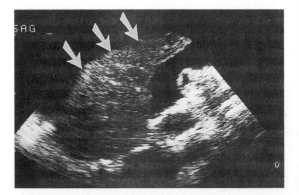

Fig. 24-1. *Ultrasound of the liver shows a highly echogenic liver with scalloped margins (arrows) surrounded by areas of decreased echogenicity. These findings were interpreted as showing a cirrhotic liver surrounded by ascites fluid.*

DISCUSSION

rhosis. The hepatitis B virus has major antigens on the surface of the viral particle and in its core. The presence of immunoglobulin directed against hepatitis B surface antigen indicates an immunological response to the virus. The response usually is not effective at cleaning the body of viral particles because only the surface protein is bound and the core remains infective. The presence of hepatitis B core antigen indicates an active infection in which viral precursors are present.

4. Serious infection such as pneumonia places a metabolic strain on the liver since many toxins must be cleared. This strain is reflected in an exacerbation of the hepatic disease that leads to increased serum bilirubin levels. Dilation of esophageal veins in response to portal hypertension produces esophageal varices. The varices are dangerous because their rupture may lead to massive gastrointestinal bleeding and death. Part of the pathophysiology of chronic active hepatitis appears to involve autoimmune processes. Steroid therapy may consequently ameliorate the process. Lactulose and neomycin are used to prevent or ameliorate the neurological dysfunction associated with severe hepatic dysfunction. The insoluble antibiotic neomycin reduces the metabolic load associated with bacterial overgrowth of the gut. The nonabsorbable disaccharide lactulose produces a mild diarrhea. It also tends to ameliorate hepatic encephalopathy by trapping ammonia in the gut.

5. The incidence of serious infection of the graft with hepatitis B virus is sufficiently low that patients with a history of hepatitis B infection are still considered suitable transplant candidates at some clinical institutions. The patient's lethargy probably reflects a toxic metabolic state. *Scleral icterus* is the term used for the discoloration of the sclera of the eye produced by hyperbilirubinemia.

6. Increased prothrombin and partial thromboplastin times probably reflected a coagulopathy secondary to inadequate synthesis of clotting factors by the liver. Stools containing occult blood suggest either oozing blood in the gastrointestinal tract or acute bleeding secondary to portal hypertension. However, other possible gastrointestinal sources of bleeding, such as a tumor or an ulcer, should also be considered. Splenomegaly occurs when splenic sinusoids dilate secondary to chronic portal hypertension. Splenomegaly usually precedes the formation of esophageal varices. Severely

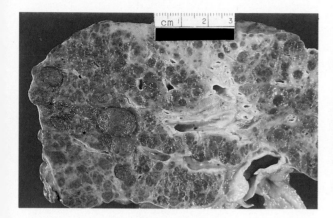

Fig. 24-2. Macronodular cirrhosis (gross photograph). The liver shows bile-tinged nodules of various sizes. This macronodular cirrhosis was accompanied by massive ascites, jaundice, hepatic failure, splenomegaly, and esophageal varices. This patient's macronodular cirrhosis is secondary to infection with hepatitis B virus.

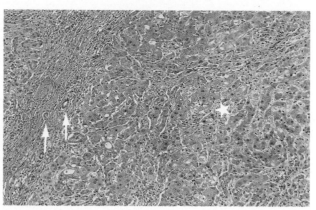

Fig. 24-3. Chronic active hepatitis B infection (low power photomicrograph, hematoxylin and eosin). Persistent hepatitis B infection has caused a disruption of the normal hepatic architecture. Cholestasis, indicated by yellowish staining of tissue, has caused atrophy and death of some hepatocytes *(asterisk)*. Bile duct proliferation *(arrows)* is seen in areas of fibrosis.

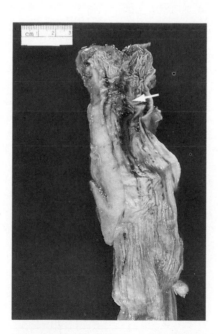

Fig. 24-4. Esophageal erosion (gross photograph). The esophagus shows a large area of erosion *(arrow)*, which may have been the source of the massive gastrointestinal hemorrhage that led to the patient's death.

CASE

One week after admission, the patient's platelet count was 19,000/mm³ (normal, 150,000 to 450,000/mm³). Her condition was relatively stable for the next five days, after which she began to experience intermittent oozing of blood from her nose. An increasing coagulopathy was followed by significant gastrointestinal bleeding. The patient was transferred to an intensive care unit.[7] Her blood pressure fell to 100/80 mmHg with a pulse of 92/min. The hematocrit was 19.6% (normal, 35 to 47%). A nasogastric tube returned bright red blood, which did not clear despite lavage. The patient aspirated a large amount of blood. She was intubated. Despite vigorous resuscitation, she sustained a cardiopulmonary arrest and was pronounced dead.[8]

Autopsy results showed active macronodular cirrhosis with hepatic failure, esophageal varices, massive ascites, and splenomegaly (Figs. 24-2 and 24-3). The gastrointestinal tract from the esophagus to the colon was massively distended and contained several liters of partially coagulated blood. The specific source of the massive acute gastrointestinal hemorrhage was not identified, but an eroded area in the esophagus appeared most likely (Fig. 24-4). Gross or microscopic hemorrhage was observed in the skin, lungs, kidneys, and esophagus. The bone marrow contained reduced numbers of megakaryocytes. The brain showed mild, icteric discoloration of the dura mater and gliosis involving the globus pallidus, substantia nigra, and inferior olivary nucleus. This gliosis was considered to be related to the history of chronic liver disease. Massive hemorrhage from esophageal varices was considered the probable cause of death.

DISCUSSION

cirrhotic livers are usually small because of the retraction produced as the fibrotic tissue matures.

7. The reason for this patient's very low platelet count was not completely clear, but several factors may have contributed. Depleted serum clotting factors sometimes cause multiple tiny hemorrhages throughout the body, in particular in the gut. The plugging of such hemorrhages may consume large numbers of platelets. Also, the prednisone and/or the patient's toxic metabolic state may have led to failure of the bone marrow to produce platelets. Furthermore, hepatic failure can cause a modest degree of bone marrow suppression, probably secondary to accumulated toxins. Alternatively, decreased synthesis of erythropoietin by kidneys affected by hepatic toxicity may have contributed to decreased platelet production.

8. An abrupt decrease in blood pressure, accompanied by an increased heart rate, can be caused by a process such as hemorrhage, massive pulmonary embolism, myocardial infarction, or septic shock. Continued bleeding is indicated by the continuing bloody fluid returned by lavage of the stomach. In addition to the obvious danger of exsanguination, bleeding by esophageal varices is dangerous because blood is a strong stomach irritant and can cause vomiting with risk of aspiration of blood.

9. In active macronodular cirrhosis, the liver attempts to regenerate and produces nodules varying from microscopic to several inches in diameter. The pattern is typically produced by processes such as viral and autoimmune disease, in contrast to the micronodular pattern produced by alcoholism. The reduced number of megakaryocytes indicates that bone marrow suppression, possibly as a result of prednisone therapy, contributed to the patient's thrombocytopenia with subsequent hemorrhage into many tissues. Specific sites of hemorrhage are often difficult to identify at autopsy because the lesion may be small and the vessels usually collapse after death and because large volumes of clotted blood may obscure organ surfaces.

Hepatic Cirrhosis

The liver is a complex organ, and disruption of its structures has widespread physiological consequences. If the biliary system is disrupted by scarring, it may not be possible for bile to enter the bile ducts and be secreted into the duodenum. This may disrupt digestion of fat, since bile salts aid the formation of lipid micelles. Also, compounds that would normally be secreted into the bile, notably the bile pigment bilirubin, instead enter the bloodstream in increased quantities. This process leads to increased serum bilirubin levels and is visible clinically as jaundice. A yellow tinge to the sclera of the eye (scleral icterus) may be visible before skin discoloration becomes prominent. Cirrhosis can also disrupt the sinusoids and larger vessels in the liver. Such disruption leads to portal hypertension and all of its possible sequelae. The spleen enlarges because of the back pressure on its outflow. Hemorrhoids, esophageal varices, and prominent abdominal venous markings are produced as alternative channels for blood flow begin to dilate.

The liver is a major synthesizer of several serum proteins. If enough liver cells die, the liver may not be able to synthesize adequate quantities of these proteins. Serum albumin levels may drop, leading to reduced serum oncotic pressure, which in turn potentially produces ascites, systemic edema, and pulmonary edema. Serum levels of many of the proteins in the clotting cascade may also be diminished, leading to potentially serious coagulopathy. Such coagulopathy can be observed clinically by monitoring the increase in prothrombin and partial thromboplastin times. The liver is the major detoxifier of many compounds and the major producer of urea from nitrogenous compounds. When too much liver tissue dies, these functions can no longer be adequately performed. Toxic metabolic states, potentially leading to depressed consciousness and coma, develop. The ability of the liver to perform these roles can be observed clinically by monitoring the blood ammonia level. The cirrhotic liver is also at increased risk for hepatocellular cancer, probably because of the risk associated with repeated regeneration of hepatic tissue.

Questions

1. How did this woman acquire hepatitis? Describe the progression of her liver disease. What problems did she experience that were directly related to her liver disease?
2. Describe this patient's hospital course. How did she die? What was found at autopsy?
3. Why do esophageal varices develop following hepatic cirrhosis? Why are they dangerous? What effects does hepatic disease have on homeostasis? How does this exacerbate the problem of bleeding esophageal varices?

Selected Reading

Achard JL: Cirrhosis of the liver: new concepts. Compr Ther 15:11–16, 1989.

Bruckstein AH: Chronic hepatitis. The challenge of diagnosis and treatment. Postgrad Med 85:67–74, 1989.

Burnett DA, Rikkers LF: Nonoperative treatment of variceal hemorrhage. Surg Clin N Am 70:291–306, 1990.

URINARY
SYSTEM

25 RENAL TRANSPLANT IN A PATIENT WITH POLYCYSTIC KIDNEY DISEASE

Key Words | polycystic kidney disease, renal failure, renal transplant, surgical complications

CASE

The patient was a 49-year-old man with end-stage renal disease, secondary to polycystic kidney disease (Fig. 25-1). His mother and one brother had died of renal complications.[1] He had known about his kidney disease for more than 20 years and had longstanding hypertension.[2] He was noted to be in renal failure when aged 48, but refused to start dialysis for eight months. He then presented with uremic pericarditis, which necessitated pericardiocentesis. He began hemodialysis by using an arteriovenous fistula; one month later he was switched to peritoneal dialysis through a dialysis catheter. He did well, without peritonitis or catheter tract infection but with little urine output, for 11 months.[3]

The patient was then readmitted for cadaveric kidney transplant. His blood urea nitrogen was 64 mg/100 ml (normal, 6 to 20 mg/100 ml) and his serum creatinine was 19.2 mg/100 ml (normal, 0.5 to 1.4 mg/100 ml). Results of other laboratory studies were not remarkable. Transplantation of a cadaveric kidney was performed on the day after admission. The transplanted kidney was located in the right lumbar region, and both of the original kidneys were left in place. The surgery ap-

DISCUSSION

1. A rare autosomal recessive form of polycystic kidney disease is characterized by bilaterally enlarged kidneys containing multiple fusiform cysts oriented radially. This disease typically causes death in infancy. An autosomal dominant adult polycystic kidney disease, such as this patient had, is more common and may be completely asymptomatic until midlife. It is also characterized by bilaterally enlarged kidneys, but the cysts are round rather than fusiform and may completely replace the renal parenchyma. In the early stages of life, the cysts are small and involve only a small percentage of the kidney. Later, they slowly enlarge and compromise renal function. The cysts are usually lined by renal tubular epithelium.

2. Hypertension and progressive chronic anemia are typical presenting complaints in patients with polycystic kidney disease. The patient's hypertension is probably secondary to increased renin secretion since the fluid-filled cystic spaces in the polycystic kidney probably impair glomerular perfusion even before renal function has been markedly diminished by destruction of glomeruli. The anemia is the result of decreased erythropoietin synthesis by the diseased kidney.

3. There are usually long intervals between diagnosis of

CASE

peared to be without complications. Nursing notes indicated that the patient was found not breathing by a nurse's aide 16 hours after surgery. He died in spite of all resuscitation measures, including open heart massage.[4]

The autopsy revealed a large retroperitoneal hematoma around the transplanted kidney. It was thought to represent the hemorrhage of approximately 4 to 6 units of blood. A specific bleeding source could not be found within this mass of blood, but the arterial and venous anastomoses were intact. Since some of the hemorrhage was subcapsular near the renal hilum, and since the hilum was at the center of the hematoma, it appeared likely that the hemorrhage originated from a subcapsular vessel near the hilum.[5] Microscopic examination of the transplanted kidney showed foci of tubular necrosis. Also, areas of wavy fibers were present in the left ventricular myocardium.[6] The autopsy also showed very severe coronary artery disease with cardiomegaly and an old myocardial infarct (Fig. 25-2). The liver showed focal areas of cystic change consistent with polycystic disease (Fig. 25-3).[7]

The patient's original kidneys were not removed during surgery. They were found at autopsy to be markedly enlarged (right, 4 lb [1,800 g]; left, 3.3 lb [1,500 g]) and to have multiple cysts containing clear brown fluid (Fig. 25-4). The cysts varied in size from 1 to 5 cm in the greatest dimen-

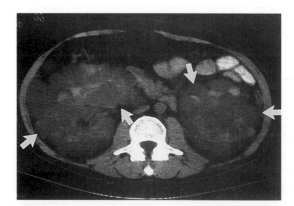

Fig. 25-1. Computed tomography of the abdomen shows bilaterally enlarged kidneys filled with multiple round cysts *(arrows)*.

DISCUSSION

the disease (often as the incidental finding of enlarged kidneys during physical examination, ultrasonography, or radiological studies) and development of renal failure sufficiently severe to require dialysis. The prospect of long-term dialysis is sufficiently intimidating that it is not uncommon for patients to resist starting dialysis until prominent complications develop. Pericarditis can develop in the presence of uremia, probably as a result of accumulated metabolic toxins. Pericardiocentesis removes accumulated fluid from the pericardial sac. In hemodialysis, the blood is pumped out of an artery and through an artificial kidney machine that contains a dialysis membrane with dialysate fluid on the other side. In peritoneal dialysis, the dialysis fluid is introduced into the peritoneal cavity and the peritoneum acts as the dialyzing membrane. Infection is a major risk in any procedure in which a catheter is placed through the skin into an organ, vessel, or body space.

4. Peritoneal dialysis does not usually restore blood urea nitrogen and creatinine levels to normal, although it does reduce them. In renal transplantation, the native kidneys are left in place to simplify surgery. They may also still provide modest degrees of renal function. Many transplanted kidneys are placed within the bony pelvis, where they are better protected. Others, as in this case, are placed in the lumbar region. The kidneys are often stabilized by being attached to adjacent structures with staples or sutures. Although transplantation of a kidney is often performed without complications, death can occur. After an apparently uneventful surgery and early recovery period, this patient was suddenly found dead or near death, and resuscitation was not possible.

5. Autopsy revealed that the cause of death was massive hemorrhage around the transplanted kidney. Interestingly, the patient appeared to have bled not from the surgical anastomoses attaching the cadaveric kidney to his arterial and venous system, but from an unidentified subcapsular artery near the renal hilum that might have been damaged during the transplantation procedures. It is often difficult to identify a specific site of bleeding in a large hematoma because the vessels collapse after death and the clot encases all of the involved structures. This is particularly true when the bleeding was a diffuse oozing rather than a flow from a single well-defined site.

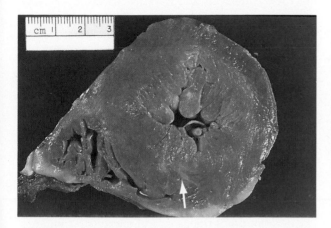

Fig. 25-2. Left ventricular hypertrophy (gross photograph). The left ventricular wall is so massively hypertrophied that the chamber lumen *(center)* is only a small fraction of its normal size. The hypertrophy may have been unrelated to the patient's hypertension. Despite the mass of muscular tissue, this heart was probably not an efficient pump because its stroke volume would have been very small. Whitish areas of fibrosis *(arrow)* are probably old infarctions.

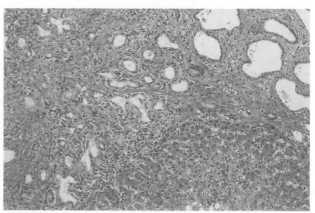

Fig. 25-3. Polycystic kidney disease involving the liver (low power photomicrograph, hematoxylin and eosin). A hepatic lobule is present in the lower right corner of the field. Multiple cysts of various sizes are present. The lining of these cysts resembles that of the intrahepatic bile ducts.

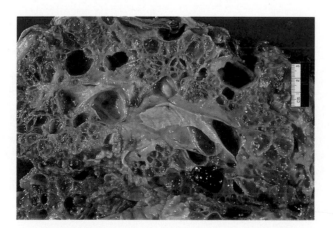

Fig. 25-4. Polycystic kidney (gross photograph). The renal parenchyma of this large polycystic kidney is almost completely replaced by cysts of various sizes. Such kidneys may cause no symptoms for many years. Pain and localized tenderness can occur when cysts are infected or hemorrhagic.

CASE

sion. The intervening stroma was fibrotic, but with some normal renal parenchyma present. Microscopically, the cysts were lined by a cuboidal to low columnar epithelium. Some cysts contained homogeneous pink material. The septae contained atrophic glomeruli, tubules, and vessels with chronic inflammation, fibrosis, and focal calcification.[8]

DISCUSSION

6. The tubular necrosis and wavy myocardial fibers indicate that there was a period of ischemia 8 to 12 hours before the patient's death, which may have been the time when the bleeding became severe. It is possible that continued careful postoperative observation would have identified a dropping blood pressure late after surgery that might have permitted transfusions and emergency surgery to correct the bleeding problem before it caused the patient's death.
7. The coronary artery disease and myocardial infarct are evidence of a longstanding defect in cardiac muscle oxygenation. Polycystic disease often involves the liver as well as the kidneys. In most patients, the liver disease is less extensive than the renal disease.
8. The description of the gross and microscopic findings in the patient's original kidneys are typical of adult polycystic kidney disease. The normal weight of a kidney is approximately .33 lb (150 g).

Chronic Renal Failure

Chronic renal failure is the end result of many kidney diseases and is characterized by loss of the functions supplied by the kidney. As the effective renal blood flow drops, serum creatinine and urea levels rise. Markedly decreased, or even absent, urine output is typical of most forms of chronic renal disease and secondarily causes fluid and sodium retention with resulting edema. In a few forms of renal failure, dehydration can occur early in the renal disease as a result of impairment of renal concentrating ability, leading to excretion of large volumes of urine.

Once renal failure develops, many other organ systems can be secondarily affected. High blood urea content (azotemia) causes generalized symptoms such as fatigue, weakness, and malaise. Gastrointestinal symptoms include a metallic taste, anorexia, nausea, and morning vomiting. A wide variety of neuromuscular symptoms can also occur; these include symptoms of peripheral neuropathy such as paresthesias, fatigue, muscle cramps, and myoclonic jerks. Itching is also a prominent symptom. Failure of tubular excretion of hydrogen ions leads to metabolic acidosis. Failure of

erythropoietin production leads to normochromic, normocytic anemia. Reduced renal blood flow leads to hypertension. Failure of the activation of vitamin D leads to renal osteodystrophy. Platelet function is also often abnormal.

Restriction of dietary protein will at least temporarily control many symptoms of renal failure by limiting the quantities of protein catabolites that are produced. When renal failure, of whatever cause, becomes sufficiently severe, it is necessary that the kidney's excretory function be performed by some other structure. Techniques commonly used for definitive therapy are hemodialysis, peritoneal dialysis, and kidney transplantation.

Questions

1. What is polycystic kidney disease? What is the probable relationship between polycystic kidney disease and hypertension? Why does polycystic kidney disease cause chronic anemia? Which other organ can also have cystic changes in a patient with polycystic disease? In most patients, which organ is more severely affected?

2. What is chronic renal failure? In what ways can chronic renal failure affect other organ systems? What problems did this patient experience? How is chronic renal failure treated?

3. What complications might occur during renal transplantation surgery? How would you recognize that a complication might be occurring? In what ways might you intervene? What happened to this patient? What was found at autopsy?

Selected Reading

Gabow PA, Schrier RW: Pathophysiology of adult polycystic kidney disease. Adv Nephrol 18:19–32, 1989.

Land W: Kidney transplantation — state of the art. Transplant Proc 21:1425–1429, 1989.

Waxman K: Postoperative multiple organ failure. Crit Care Clin 3:429–440, 1987.

CASE

plaints may have been related to the extensive studding of the small intestine with tumors. Her severe hypoxia was probably the result of tumor emboli with thrombosis, causing occlusion of multiple small arteries within the lungs (Figs. 26-2 and 26-3). This process also led to pulmonary infarction. Her lymphoma was apparently in complete remission at the time of her death. Review of the autopsy slides of this case during the preparation of this book suggested that the tumor cells resembled squamous epithelium more than transitional epithelium. This observation raised the possibility that the tumor was cervical cancer that had extended into the bladder rather than the transitional cell cancer that had been diagnosed.[10]

DISCUSSION

patient's death, they were not the typical emboli related to deep venous thrombosis. Rather, tumor emboli were trapped in the lung and formed a surface for thrombosis. This thrombosis may have suddenly reached a critical point at which pulmonary infarction and the patient's severe hypoxia developed. The *Klebsiella* pneumonia may also have contributed to her death. Infection is common in cancer patients and can be unsuspected because the patient's symptoms are attributed to the tumor. The question about the histological type of the tumor reminds the reader to remember that errors and areas of controversy can occur in anatomic pathology.

Lymphomas

Lymphomas can be considered neoplasms of the immune system. Malignant transformation can occur at any stage in the differentiation of B and T lymphocytes. Also included among the lymphomas are tumorous transformations of an unproven cell line, possibly one of the structural cells present in lymph nodes, that produce Hodgkin's disease. These neoplastic disorders are clinically and pathologically diverse. The cells in non-Hodgkin's lymphomas can be large or small, can have cleaved or uncleaved nuclei, and can be arranged in diffuse or follicular patterns. This diversity has led to the development of several classification schemes whose intent is to provide subclasses of lymphomas that have a more homogeneous prognosis and clinical behavior, with the possible implication of a more homogeneous response to therapy. The description of these various classification schemes is beyond the scope of this discussion, but can be found in standard internal medicine, pathology, and hematology texts.

The complications and clinical manifestations of lymphoma have a variety of origins. Enlarging lymph nodes can compress adjacent structures. Depending upon the location of the nodes, such structures include airways, blood vessels, the gastrointestinal tract and its related organs, and the urinary tract. Infiltration of adjacent tissue also occurs and can lead to ulceration or perforation of the gastrointestinal tract and pneumonia in the lungs. Lymphoma involvement in the central nervous system can cause symptoms of cord compression and occasionally meningitis. Bone marrow involvement may produce anemia, neutropenia, and thrombocytopenia. Hyperuricemia may be present and may be exacerbated by the cell death caused by effective chemotherapy. Second malignancies also occur after both chemotherapy and radiation therapy.

Questions

1. What is a lymphoma? How did this patient's lymphoma present? How was it diagnosed and treated? How successful was the therapy?
2. What clinical manifestations led to the discovery in this patient of tumor involving the bladder? How was her tumor diagnosed and treated? What intestinal and urinary tract complications did she experience? How were these related to her disease?

3. How did this patient die? What evidence of pulmonary disease was found at autopsy? How did her tumor contribute to her death? What was the status of her lymphoma at the time of her death?

Selected Reading

Lecart C: Cervical cancer. Epidemiology, histopathology, diagnosis. J Belge Radiol 71:383–392, 1988.

Raghaven D, Shipley WU, Garnick MB et al: Biology and management of bladder cancer. N Engl J Med 322:1129–1138, 1990.

27 ACUTE RENAL FAILURE SECONDARY TO LYMPHOMA

Key Words | lymphoma, hydronephrosis, acute renal failure

CASE

A 75-year-old man presented to a community hospital emergency room with complaints of markedly increased lower extremity edema. The patient reported having produced only small volumes of urine in the preceding several days. His blood urea nitrogen was 122 mg/100 ml (normal, 6 to 20 mg/100 ml), and his creatinine was 11.5 mg/100 ml (normal, 0.5 to 1.4 mg/100 ml). A renal ultrasonogram showed a small left kidney and marked hydronephrosis on the right.[1] A stent was placed on the right, and the patient's creatinine decreased slightly but then rose again. The stent was removed, and the patient was transferred to the renal service of a university hospital.[2]

Pyelogram studies performed after the transfer showed a dilated pelvis and dilated calyces in the right kidney. The exact site of obstruction could not be determined, but the right ureter was slightly dilated to the level of spinal vertebra S-1. The left kidney showed a normal collecting system. The left ureter did not fill. The impression was that the patient probably had a retroperitoneal tumor, most probably lymphoma obstructing his ureters. The patient was thought to need bilateral stent placement. This was performed the following day, after he had been treated with dialysis to improve his metabolic status.[3] He had a brisk postoperative diuresis. His serum creatinine decreased, reaching 1.9 mg/100 ml after several

DISCUSSION

1. Lower extremity edema can be due to a variety of processes including renal or cardiac failure, obstruction of lymphatics, or local processes involving the lower extremities. Failure to produce urine suggests that acute renal failure may be occurring. The patient's azotemia, or high blood urea nitrogen and creatine levels, suggests that he needed prompt treatment since his kidneys were functioning inadequately. *Hydronephrosis* refers to dilation of the renal pelvis and calyces by urine. It typically occurs when the ureter has been partially obstructed for a prolonged period, causing urine to accumulate without draining adequately into the bladder. In contrast, rapid, complete obstruction of a ureter can cause renal shutdown without causing hydronephrosis. The finding of hydronephrosis suggests that this patient's acute renal failure may be secondary to ureteral obstruction. The disease processes involving the left kidney are less clear; a small kidney can occur as the end stage of many renal diseases.

2. A stent is a semirigid tube that is placed within a tubular body structure, such as a ureter, to ensure that the lumen remains open. Ureteral stents can be placed either during surgery or without surgery by using a cystoscope to visualize the ureteral openings on the interior surface of the bladder. The decrease in serum creatinine after stent placement suggests that renal function was at least partially restored; the subsequent rise in creatinine after the stent was removed suggests that the obstruction was not a temporary problem.

CASE

weeks. The left kidney continued to function more poorly than the right.[4]

Approximately 1 week after admission, the patient's serum creatinine had begun to stabilize. At that time, a ureterolysis with biopsy of the tumor mass was performed. The peritoneal mass was seen at surgery to extend from the right renal hilum almost to the bladder and to encase the iliac vessels and the vena cava. During surgery, the right ureter was wrapped with omentum and moved outside the retroperitoneum and into the abdomen. The frozen biopsy section showed lymphoma. A subsequent fixed section showed intermediate-grade, diffuse large cell lymphoma (Figs. 27-1 and 27-2). Immunological studies demonstrated that the tumor cells expressed B-cell markers but did not express surface immunoglobulins (Fig. 27-3).[5]

Postoperatively, the patient's course was complicated by his massive lower extremity edema, which prevented him from ambulating well. He developed pneumonia and a urinary tract infection, which required intravenous antibiotics. Several attempts were made to remove his stents, but after each removal his creatinine began to rise. Therefore the stents were replaced, and the serum creatinine decreased.[6]

A bone marrow biopsy performed two weeks after admission showed diffuse involvement with large cell lymphoma. The patient was considered to have stage 4 lymphoma and was thought to be a good candidate for chemotherapy with CHOP. Since it was thought that his therapy might best be performed near his home, he was transferred back to the community hospital. At the time of his transfer, his stents were still in place and his creatinine was 1.9 mg/100 ml. His only significant disability was his lower extremity edema. His subsequent course was lost to follow-up at the university hospital.[7]

DISCUSSION

3. Failure of the left ureter to fill during the pyelogram suggests that the left ureter was completely obstructed; since the right ureter did fill, some urine was flowing through it. Bilateral stenting potentially corrected these obstructions. The abdominal retroperitoneal lymph nodes are predominantly located near the aorta and iliac vessels. Involvement of these nodes by lymphoma can cause obstruction of the ureters, whose course runs nearby in the retroperitoneal space. In a patient requiring emergency procedures, it can sometimes be advantageous to briefly defer the procedures to partially correct severe metabolic problems, such as this patient's high urea nitrogen and creatinine levels, which were corrected by dialysis.
4. The patient's condition improved as soon as urine could flow through his ureters. The brisk diuresis occurred as a response of his now functioning kidneys to the fluid overload that had developed during the period of acute renal failure. The continued poor functioning of the left kidney suggests that it may have been more badly damaged, perhaps by a more sudden, complete, and prolonged obstruction than that which involved the right ureter.
5. Because of the size of the tumor mass, no attempt was made to remove it completely. Ureterolysis is a surgical procedure in which the ureters are dissected free of any adjacent tumor or scar tissue. Since the ureters are very delicate and can be deeply buried in a large, hard, tumor mass, ureterolysis can be a difficult and lengthy surgical procedure. The right ureter was wrapped in omentum and placed in the abdominal cavity to try to protect it from further involvement with tumor. A frozen section of a biopsy can be performed during surgery to make an initial diagnosis, but this diagnosis should always be confirmed later with sections of fixed biopsy material. Large cell lymphomas usually contain less mature cells than small cell lymphomas. The large cell lymphomas are almost always of intermediate or high grade. The term *diffuse* refers to the failure of the tumor to form distinct nodules containing germinal centers. Immunological studies are used to further characterize lymphomas. Most lymphomas are derived from B-cell lines. Some relatively mature B-cell lines will express antibody or antibody precursors on their cell surfaces.

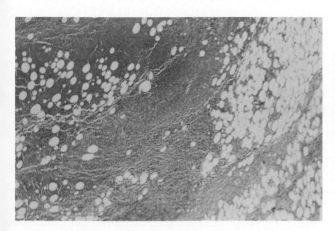

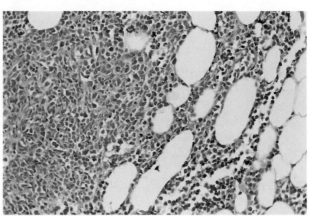

Fig. 27-1. Large cell lymphoma (low power photomicrograph, hematoxylin and eosin). This specimen shows lymphoma invading the mesenteric fat in the peritoneal cavity. The lymphoma appears as masses of dark purplish-stained cells interspersed between the clear fat cells of the mesentery. Since the germinal centers are not formed, the pattern of tumor growth is considered to be diffuse rather than nodular.

Fig. 27-2. Lymphoma, detail of Fig. 27-1 (high power photomicrograph, hematoxylin and eosin). The tumor appears as masses of cells with densely stained nuclei and scant cytoplasm.

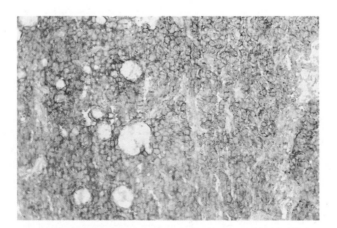

Fig. 27-3. Lymphoma stained for B-cell markers (high power photomicrograph, immunological stain for Leu-14). The entire field of cells stains positively (brown) for the B-cell marker Leu-14. This uniform staining indicates that this is a monoclonal proliferation of lymphocytes rather than a reactive lymphocytosis.

DISCUSSION

6. The persistence of the patient's severe lower extremity edema after his renal function improved suggests that it was not simply a consequence of his renal failure but, rather, may have been primarily due to obstruction by the tumor mass of the lymphatic drainage of his legs. It is common for seriously ill patients to develop additional infections while hospitalized. This patient was predisposed to pneumonia by the bed rest associated with hospitalization, and he was predisposed to urinary tract infections by the multiple procedures performed on his urinary tract, by the stent placement, and by the tumor. The failure of the attempts to remove the stents suggests that the tumor mass continued to compress the ureters and that the stents were required to keep the ureters patent.

7. Stage 4 indicates the presence of widely disseminated lymphoma. The acronym CHOP is used for combination chemotherapy with the alkylating agent cyclophosphamide (Cytoxan), the antibiotic doxorubicin (Adriamycin), the mitotic inhibitor vincristine (Oncovin), and the steroid prednisone. (The acronym is no longer a good mnemonic because of changes in drug names.) Medical staff often do not hear of a patient's course after the patient is transferred to another hospital.

Acute Renal Failure

Acute renal failure refers to a new onset of azotemia, indicated by rising blood urea nitrogen and serum creatinine levels, which is often accompanied by decreased urine output. Many diseases can cause acute renal failure. It is helpful to divide these diseases into processes that involve prerenal, renal, or postrenal structures.

Prerenal processes that can cause acute renal failure usually do so by decreasing the pressure of blood perfusing the kidney. The decrease in pressure may be systemic, as occurs in heart failure or shock following severe bacterial infection or severe hemorrhage, or may be due to local obstruction of the renal artery by processes such as an adjacent abdominal aneurysm or a tumor mass.

Severe alterations in the glomerular filtration rate can cause acute renal failure and can occur secondary to changes in renal blood flow, hydrostatic pressure, capillary oncotic pressure, or capillary permeability. Severe acute glomerulonephritis can cause acute renal failure by limiting the total glomerular filtration surface. Acute renal failure can also accompany interstitial nephritis, acute tubular necrosis, and vascular disease with the kidney.

Postrenal causes of acute renal failure principally involve bilateral obstruction of ureters, obstruction of the bladder, or obstruction of the urethra by processes such as tumor, prostate hypertrophy, stones, or compression by an external mass.

Questions

1. What is acute renal failure? What types of processes can cause acute renal failure? Give examples of typical causes of prerenal, renal, and postrenal failure.
2. How did this patient present? How was his renal problem diagnosed? What was the purpose of the stents that were placed? Were the stents successful in this patient?
3. Which process caused the patient's obstruction? De-

scribe the tumor that was found. How was the patient treated, and what further treatment was planned?

Selected Reading

Awazu M, Barakat AY, Chevalier RL, Ichikawa I: The cause of uremia in obstructed kidneys. J Pediatr 114:179–186, 1989.

Bidani A, Churchill PC: Acute renal failure. Dis Mon 35:57–132, 1989.

Skarin AT: Non-Hodgkin's lymphoma. Adv Intern Med 34:209–242, 1989.

28 RENAL DISEASE FOLLOWING ACUTE PHARYNGITIS

Key Words | glomerulonephritis, streptococci

CASE*

A 26-year old woman developed severe pharyngitis. She was seen in a convenient care center, where a throat swab test gave results that were positive for streptococci. After a five-day course of erythromycin, she reportedly felt better, but several days later she had gradual onset of nausea, weakness, and malaise. Her urine appeared dark to her, but she attributed this darkness to blood contamination secondary to her concurrent menstrual period.[1]

After several days of gradually increasing symptoms, she presented to an emergency room with gross hematuria. Her blood urea nitrogen at that time was 49 mg/100 ml (normal, 6 to 20 mg/100 ml), and her creatinine was 5.5 mg/100 ml (normal, 0.5 to 1.4 mg/100 ml). She was admitted for evaluation. Her physical examination was unremarkable. A variety of immunological studies were performed to elucidate the cause of her renal disease. Of these studies, only the ASO and AHT titers were strongly positive. A renal biopsy showed 4 of 13 glomeruli with epithelial proliferation and crescent formation. Electron microscopy

---

* Note to reader: This case is particularly complex. We include the case because we believe that seeing at least a few complicated cases in which a definitive diagnosis is never reached is an important part of a student's education.

DISCUSSION

1. Despite the common lay use of the term "strep throat," not all pharyngitis is attributable to streptococcal infection. The diagnosis is suspected when a patient presents with a severe pharyngitis, and it can be confirmed by commercially available tests for streptococcal antigen that are performed on throat swabs. The development of additional symptoms after the sore throat began to resolve suggests that a second pathological process may have been occurring. Possibilities include acquisition of a second infection and post-streptococcal syndromes such as rheumatic heart disease or post-streptococcal renal disease. Dark urine can be attributed to either increased levels of bilirubin or blood contamination.

2. Blood in the urine can come from any part of the urinary tract or from outside sources such as menstrual blood. Urea and creatinine are excreted by the kidneys, and their blood concentration increases when renal function is diminished. The combination of increasing blood urea nitrogen and serum creatinine is called *azotemia*. Anti-streptolysin O (ASO) and anti-streptococcal hyaluronidase (AHT) titers are a measure of the amount of immunoglobin directed against streptococci. An elevation of these titers suggests recent exposure to streptococcal antigens. Crescents are epithelial proliferations of the lining of Bowman's capsule, and they suggest recent severe damage to a glomerulus. Deposits seen by electron microscopy during glomerular disease are often deposits of immune com-

CASE

of the biopsy specimen showed mesangial deposits and occasional subepithelial deposits (Fig. 28-1).[2]

The patient was considered clinically to have post-streptococcal glomerulonephritis. Her renal function initially improved sufficiently for her to be discharged home without further therapy and monitored as an outpatient. Her creatinine reached a nadir of 3.6 mg/100 ml approximately one month after her pharyngitis began. The following week, it rose to 5.2 mg/100 ml, and she was readmitted. On admission, she had no new overt symptoms. Her creatinine clearance was 13 ml/min (normal, 80 to 120 ml/min). She continued to have proteinuria (2 +) and hematuria (3 +). Her total urinary protein was 3.2 g/24 h (normal, < 150 mg/24 h).[3]

Results of an open biopsy demonstrated marked progression of the glomerular disease. The disease process involving the kidneys was complex (Figs. 28-2 and 28-3). Of 160 glomeruli examined, only 1 was normal; all the others contained crescents. The renal tubules were separated by a marked inflammatory infiltrate composed of lymphocytes, plasma cells, monocytes, and occasional eosinophils. Tubules in some areas contained proteinaceous material, cellular debris, or red blood cells.[4]

Immunofluorescence studies of the biopsy specimen gave complex results with a variety of antibodies and complement factors found in glomerular crescents, tubular epithelial cells, tubular casts, and interstitium. The intact portions of the glomeruli stained positively only for complement factor C3 and properdin. Electron microscopy studies showed paramesangial deposits but no subepithelial or subendothelial deposits (Fig. 28-4).[5]

The cause of the necrotizing glomerulonephritis was not clear. The histological pattern was considered to be inconsistent with postinfectious causes and with Goodpasture syndrome. Vasculitis was a strong consideration, although arteritis was not seen on biopsy. The patient's renal function deteriorated to the point that she required hemodialysis. She was treated with high-dose steroid therapy and was subsequently able to stop

DISCUSSION

plexes that either can be formed in the tissue or can be formed in the bloodstream and precipitated in the tissue.

3. This patient's case is somewhat atypical of post-streptococcal glomerulonephritis in that subepithelial electron-dense humps were not a prominent finding at renal biopsy. Improvement in renal function, usually one to two weeks after the urinary symptoms become prominent, is typical of post-streptococcal glomerulonephritis. In most patients, the glomerulonephritis resolves without sequelae. In a few, as in this patient, renal function may subsequently deteriorate following an initial improvement. Creatinine clearance is a measure of glomerular filtration rate and yields a more quantitative impression of renal function than do blood urea nitrogen or serum creatinine levels. The combination of moderate proteinuria and substantial hematuria is part of a nephritic syndrome.

4. An open biopsy is performed as a surgical procedure and permits a larger piece of tissue to be taken than is possible with a punch biopsy. Although the disease demonstrated by the first biopsy involved only some glomeruli and spared the remainder of the kidney, the second biopsy specimen demonstrated severe disease processes throughout the kidney.

5. The interpretation of immunofluorescence studies on a severely damaged kidney is difficult because it may be difficult to distinguish primary from secondary immune effects. In this case, disruption of the glomeruli may have led to a diffuse deposition in the renal tubules of many serum proteins, including antibodies and complement factors. Properdin is a serum protein in the alternate complement pathway that is activated by gram-negative bacteria in combination with antibody-antigen complexes. Staining of relatively intact portions of the glomerular capillary beds with C3 and properdin suggests that activation of the complement pathway may have been involved as an early step in the glomerular disease. The immunofluorescence staining in the interstitium was probably related to the marked inflammatory infiltrate. Prominent subepithelial electron-dense deposits would have been consistent with post-streptococcal glomerulonephritis; mesangial deposits are a nonspecific finding seen in many glomerular diseases.

6. Goodpasture syndrome is a cause of acute glomerulo-

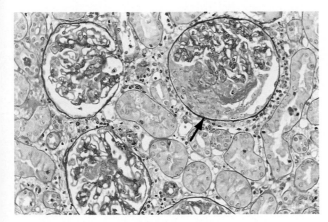

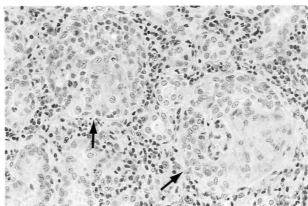

Fig. 28-1. First renal biopsy (high power photomicrograph, periodic acid-Schiff stain). This specimen was taken about two weeks after the patient's initial pharyngitis. The two glomeruli on the left appear almost normal. Slight thickening of basement membranes is the only change appreciable by light microscopy. The glomerulus on the right has crescenteric proliferation of cells within Bowman's capsule *(arrow)*. The tubules and interstitium appear healthy.

Fig. 28-2. Second renal biopsy (high power photomicrograph, hematoxylin and eosin). This specimen was taken about two months after the patient's pharyngitis. Two glomeruli *(arrows)* are present, but there has been such a proliferation of cells, both within the tufts and in Bowman's capsule, that the glomerular capillary beds are no longer recognizable. The interstitium has also been damaged and contains many more nuclei than in Fig. 28-1.

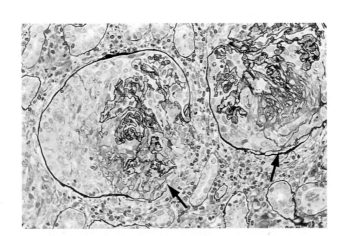

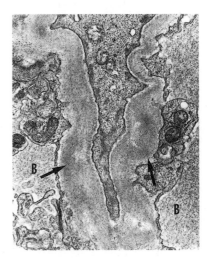

Fig. 28-3. Second renal biopsy (high power photomicrograph, Jones stain). The general appearance with this stain is similar to that illustrated in Fig. 28-1, but the basement membrane stains black rather than red. This specimen was taken from the same biopsy as Fig. 28-2 and shows a similar histological field. Here, the basement membrane bounding Bowman's capsule is both interrupted and doubled *(arrows)*. The basement membranes of the capillary tufts are displaced and compressed by extensive crescent formation. These badly compressed capillaries do not permit perfusion of the glomerular tufts.

Fig. 28-4. Glomerulonephritis (electronmicrograph). Electron-dense deposits *(arrows)* widen the subepithelial basement membrane. Spaces contiguous with the space within Bowman's capsule are indicated by the letter B.

CASE

dialysis, although her serum creatinine remained relatively high. Despite her renal condition, she was later able to become pregnant with and then deliver healthy twins.[6]

DISCUSSION

nephritis with prominent hematuria; it is caused by antibodies directed against the basement membrane of the glomerular capillaries. *Vasculitis* means an inflammation of blood vessels; it can be caused by a variety of autoimmune diseases. The diagnosis suggested by a patient's clinical history often, but not always, agrees with the diagnosis suggested by histopathology. Renal glomerular diseases are particularly notorious for sometimes producing such complex abnormalities that the cause of disease is obscured. Severe glomerular disease that has autoimmune features will sometimes, as in this patient, respond to high dose steroids. This patient recovered sufficiently to carry twins to term. However, she can be expected to continue to have less than normal renal function throughout her life, and she may eventually require frequent hemodialysis.

Post-Streptococcal Glomerulonephritis

Acute post-streptococcal glomerulonephritis can follow pharyngeal or cutaneous infection with some strains of group A β-hemolytic streptococci. Typically, nephritic syndrome develops after a latency period of one to two weeks. Clinical findings can include hematuria, proteinuria, and azotemia. In most patients, there is a spontaneous resolution of symptoms within one week of onset of the illness. In a small percentage, the illness does not resolve but instead follows a progressive course leading to chronic renal failure.

The disease processes in post-streptococcal glomerulonephritis appear to be related to deposition of circulating immune complexes within the kidney. In the typical case of post-streptococcal glomerulonephritis, focal electron-dense protein deposits, called *humps*, are found between the capillary basement membrane and the epithelial cells covering the glomerular tufts. Deposits can also be found in the glomerular mesangium. The deposits typically contain IgG, complement factor C3, and properdin. Perhaps as a response to the deposits, glomerular tufts enlarge as the cells in the mesangium and capillary endothelium proliferate. Pro-

liferation of the capillary endothelial cells can lead to partial or complete obstruction of some tuft capillaries. Significant deposition of debris and cellular proliferation within Bowman's capsule, known as glomerular crescent formation, is uncommon except in the small percentage of patients who exhibit rapidly progressive renal failure.

Questions

1. How did this patient present? What was the significance of her pharyngitis? What features of clinical picture suggested that her pharyngitis had not resolved without sequelae?
2. What clinical features suggested that this patient had developed renal disease? What is glomerulonephritis? How does it present?
3. What types of diagnoses were considered for this patient's renal disease? What was she thought to have? Discuss the results of her two biopsies. What is the significance of the difference between the two biopsies?

Selected Reading

Ayoub EM, Chun CS: Nonsuppurative complications of group A streptococcal infection. Adv Pediatr Infect Dis 5:69–92, 1990.

Bidani A, Churchill PC: Acute renal failure. Dis Mon 35:57–132, 1989.

Rosenfeld JA: Renal disease and pregnancy. Am Fam Physician 39:209–212, 1989.

NERVOUS SYSTEM

29 AMYOTROPHIC LATERAL SCLEROSIS

Key Words | amyotrophic lateral sclerosis, paralysis, degenerative neurological disease

CASE

The patient was a 62-year-old woman who had begun to experience insidious onset of left lower leg weakness five years previously. These symptoms worsened, and the evaluation of the problem included computed tomography, myelography, and electromyography. A year later, she was diagnosed as having amyotrophic lateral sclerosis.[1] Two years after onset of symptoms in her left leg, she developed right lower leg weakness. By three years after onset, she was confined to a wheelchair. Over the next one and one-half years, her trunk and neck muscles began to be affected. Her bladder and bowel control were normal. During the six months before her final admission, her symptoms had progressed particularly rapidly and she had begun to have increasing difficulty with speech and swallowing. She had become completely bedridden. Her repeated difficulties with aspiration led to admission to a hospital.[2]

The patient did not have any other medical problems. Her family history was negative for amyotrophic lateral sclerosis. She appeared cachetic, anxious, and seriously debilitated. With the exception of her neurological examination, the results of most of her physical examination were within normal limits.[3] The neurological examination showed that she was alert and oriented, but unable to speak intelligibly. All cranial nerves except IX and X, which could not be examined, appeared to be intact. Motor examination showed

DISCUSSION

1. Lower leg weakness may be due to either neurological or muscular disease with a variety of causes. *Myelography* is the radiographic study of the spinal cord. Both computed tomograms and myelograms might have revealed a mass or other lesion in the spinal nerve roots or cord that would have explained the muscle weakness. In electromyography, the nerve supplying a muscle is electrically stimulated and the evoked electrical activity in the muscle is recorded. Electromyograms are sometimes helpful in distinguishing neurological from muscular disorders and may give further information that helps to define the type of muscular disorder, if one is present. It is not uncommon for diagnosis of a neuromuscular disorder to take months to years, since the diagnosis often depends upon the pattern of progression of symptoms.

2. This patient's clinical history is typical of amyotrophic lateral sclerosis. In this disease, the neurons in the ventral horn of the spinal cord which innervate skeletal muscle slowly begin to die. This loss of cells causes a degeneration atrophy of muscles, leading progressively to weakness, paralysis, and finally a loss of deep tendon reflexes. The loss of deep tendon reflexes occurs later than the paralysis because the reflexes usually persist until denervation atrophy of the muscles progresses to the point the muscle can no longer contract. The loss of motor neurons begins in the lumbar and sacral regions and progresses cranially. Bladder and bowel control are characteristically preserved, indicating that the autonomic innervation of

181

CASE

flaccid paralysis of the right arm and both legs. The left arm was profoundly weak, with more severe involvement of proximal muscles. Sensory examination was intact throughout to light touch, pinprick, and proprioception. Deep tendon reflexes were present and normal in both arms and were completely absent in both legs. Cerebellar function was not testable. All laboratory data obtained on admission were within normal limits.[4]

The clinical impression was a patient with end-stage amyotrophic lateral sclerosis whose nutritional status was considered to be quite poor. One week after admission, a feeding gastrostomy was placed that was well tolerated postoperatively. Discharge to a hospice was planned.[5] However, on the fourth postoperative day, the patient was observed to be markedly dyspneic. Over the next several hours, her respiratory status rapidly declined. She became cyanotic, her respirations ceased, and she died. No cardiopulmonary measures were instituted.[6]

The cause of death was considered to be respiratory failure secondary to amyotrophic lateral sclerosis. The neuropathological findings showed thin and flattened ventral roots of the spinal cord and marked loss of spinal cord anterior horn cells associated with astrocytosis. There was marked demyelination and endoneurial fibrosis of anterior roots and an asymmetry in the paucity of neuronal population between one anterior horn and the other (Figs. 29-1 and 29-2). The nucleus of Oronofrowicz was preserved.[7] In the medulla oblongata, there was astrocytosis and a decrease in the number of neurons at the level of the ninth and twelfth cranial nerve nuclei. The skeletal muscles were diffusely atrophic, which was most pronounced in the lower extremities. Microscopically, the skeletal muscle was characterized by severe neurogenic atrophy (Fig. 29-3).[8]

DISCUSSION

smooth muscle is not impaired. The cranial nerve motor nuclei, which are physiological counterparts of ventral horn nuclei, become involved late in the disease. Extraocular movements characteristically remain intact, possibly because nuclei involving motor control of respiration are usually affected first and lead to death. The difficulties with swallowing can lead to both starvation and repeated aspiration of oral or gastric contents. Such aspiration can cause severe pneumonia.

3. Some, but not all, forms of amyotrophic lateral sclerosis appear to involve a familial predisposition. With the exception of poor nutritional status because she has been unable to eat adequately, this patient's general health has been good. Such good general health is typical of amyotrophic lateral sclerosis.

4. The loss of motor neurons is very selective. Touch, pinprick, proprioception, taste, vision, hearing, and mental function remain completely intact even after the loss of motor neurons is sufficiently profound to completely paralyze the patient.

5. A feeding gastrostomy is a tube, through which food can be passed, that is surgically implanted in the stomach and passed out through the abdominal wall. The surgery was well tolerated and probably did not contribute to the patient's death.

6. Amyotrophic lateral sclerosis is a disease in which patients become increasingly entrapped in their own bodies. Death in such a situation is often welcomed by both the patients and their families, and it may be inappropriate to vigorously resuscitate these patients once respiratory failure occurs.

7. Respiratory failure is a common cause of death in patients with amyotrophic lateral sclerosis and may, as in this patient, occur over a relatively brief period. In some patients, aspiration pneumonia is a cause of death. Neuropathological findings at autopsy confirm the loss of anterior horn cells and their replacement by increased numbers of astrocytes. This is the central nervous system equivalent of formation of a fibrotic scar. Death of the neurons leads to loss of tissue and to fibrosis in the ventral roots that had originally contained the motor neurons. The demyelination reflects a selective preservation of nonmyelinated axons that arise from neurons other than motor neurons. The loss is visible macroscopically as thinned and flattened ventral roots. Loss of innervation leads to atrophy of

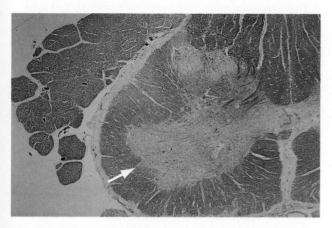

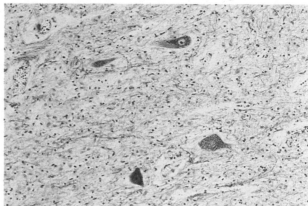

Fig. 29-1. Spinal cord in amyotrophic lateral sclerosis (low power photomicrograph, hematoxylin and eosin). The spinal cord is almost completely depleted of the large alpha motor neurons usually present in the ventral horn *(arrow)*. Loss of these neurons tends to occur first in the lumbar and sacral cord and then later progresses to higher spinal levels. The neuronal loss is accompanied by paralysis that begins in the legs and later extends to the trunk and arms.

Fig. 29-2. Spinal cord in amyotrophic lateral sclerosis, detail of Fig. 29-1 (high power photomicrograph, hematoxylin and eosin). This image shows the only four surviving alpha motor neurons from the section of spinal cord shown in the previous image. Even these few remaining cells are not normal: their cytoplasm shows an increase in darkly stained granular material compared with normal neurons.

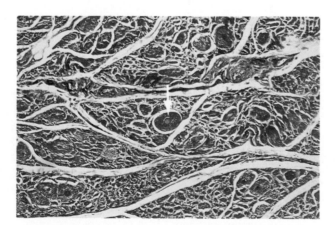

Fig. 29-3. Skeletal muscle showing denervation atrophy (high power photomicrograph, trichrome stain). Loss of innervation of skeletal muscle leads to a reduction in the size of denervated muscle fibers accompanied by hypertrophy of fibers that remain innervated. The result is a wide range of fiber sizes, such as illustrated in this field. Also present are abnormal fibers *(arrow)*, termed "target fibers," which can be found in denervated muscle.

DISCUSSION

skeletal muscle. Although not prominent in this case, a degeneration of the neurons that give rise to the corticospinal tracts also often occurs in amyotrophic lateral sclerosis and leads to degeneration of the corticospinal tracts. In many patients, there is a deficit of upper motor neurons as well. The nucleus of Oronofrowicz is a spinal cord nucleus that is involved in motor control of the bladder. Its preservation was consistent with the patient's continued bladder control.

8. The decrease in the number of neurons in the medulla was responsible for the patient's difficulty with speech and swallowing. Muscle that experiences chronic denervation of synaptic stimulation will atrophy. Neurogenic atrophy is characterized histologically by a predominance of atrophic fibers interspersed with occasional large, regenerating fibers.

Degenerative Diseases of the Nervous System

Amyotrophic lateral sclerosis is one of many degenerative diseases of the central nervous system that are characterized by progressive loss of neurons and their axons in a particular neuroanatomical system. In each of these diseases, such loss is accompanied by loss of the functions normally supplied by the neuroanatomical system. The specific symptoms and neurological findings vary with the affected system. The events leading to neuronal loss are still almost completely unknown for most of these diseases, but are thought to possibly involve enzymatic mechanisms since most of these conditions have a strong familial character. The diseases typically affect older adults and have a slowly progressive course, and often no therapy other than palliative measures is feasible. The diseases mentioned below are only a few of these neurological diseases and are chosen to illustrate the wide variety of effects that loss of a particular neuroanatomical system can produce.

When the cerebral cortex is the predominant site of cell loss, dementias, often with aphasias, are the major manifestations. Examples of diseases with progressive cerebral cortical loss include Alzheimer's disease, which involves frontal, temporal, and parietal lobes, and Pick's disease, which selectively involves the frontal lobe. When cell populations in subcortical structures are affected, the defects tend to produce disorders of movement. Thus, loss of cells in the substantia nigra produces Parkinsonism, with muscle rigidity and poverty of movement. Loss of cells in the basal ganglia produces the bizarre movements of Huntington's chorea. Loss of cells in the cerebellum disrupts feedback mechanisms used in motor control and characteristically produces ataxia and impaired gait. Examples of such cerebellar degenerative processes include Friedreich's ataxia, in which degeneration of the spinocerebellar tracts and posterior column of the spinal cord occurs, and olivopontocerebellar atrophy, in which combined degeneration of cerebellum, olives, and pons occurs.

Questions

1. Discuss the pathophysiology of amyotrophic lateral sclerosis. What was the pattern of progression of this patient's symptoms? Was it typical for patients with amyotrophic lateral sclerosis? What complications did she experience?
2. What changes are occurring in the spinal cord as the symptoms progress? What would you expect to see if

you could take microscopic sections as a function of time from the anterior horn of the spinal cord, peripheral nerve, and skeletal muscle? Relate these predicted findings to the observed changes in muscle strength and reflex activity.

3. How would you communicate with and convey emotional support to a patient with severe amyotrophic lateral sclerosis? How would you handle your own emotional reaction? What would you tell a patient who had been recently diagnosed with amyotrophic lateral sclerosis about the disease? If a patient with an untreatable disease, or a member of the family, asks you to help the patient commit suicide, how would you respond?

Selected Reading

Braun SR: Respiratory system in amyotrophic lateral sclerosis. Neurol Clin 5:9–31, 1987.

Mitsumoto H, Hanson MR, Chad DA: Amyotrophic lateral sclerosis. Recent advances in pathogenesis and therapeutic trials. Arch Neurol 45:189–209, 1988.

Neal GD, Clarke LR: Neuromuscular disorders. Otolaryngol Clin N Am 20:195–201, 1987.

30 SUBARACHNOID HEMORRHAGE AFTER RUPTURE OF BERRY ANEURYSM

Key Words | *berry aneurysm, subarachnoid hemorrhage, medical misadventure*

CASE

A 70-year-old woman, who had previously been in good health, suddenly developed headache, nausea, and vomiting. The headache was bitemporal and started just before the nausea and vomiting. The patient was taken to an emergency room at a community hospital, where she was told that she had a viral syndrome and was sent home.[1] The following morning, the patient's daughter had difficulty in arousing her. The patient was also incoherent when she spoke. She was taken back to the emergency room, where she was evaluated by computed tomography. The scan was reportedly normal except for some edema, but, when reviewed later, showed blood in the occipital horns of the lateral ventricles and some ventricular enlargement.[2] A lumbar puncture was performed with some difficulty and showed opening pressure of 420 mmH$_2$O and bloody cerebrospinal fluid (red blood cell count, >200,000 /mm^3).[3] The patient was transferred to a university hospital after treatment with furosemide and dexamethasone.[4]

The patient was lethargic. She knew her name, but did not know the date or her location. The

DISCUSSION

1. Viral syndromes are a common cause of nonspecific symptoms such as nausea, vomiting, and headache. However, it can be dangerous to simply assume that this is the problem in a patient who presents to the emergency room. Although the headache, nausea, and vomiting associated with subarachnoid hemorrhage are nonspecific, they tend to be more severe than those associated with "the flu." The fact that the patient's family was sufficiently concerned to take her to an emergency room should have suggested that the symptoms deserved adequate evaluation.

2. Neurological signs following an apparently benign condition are of grave concern and suggest that the patient's illness has not been fully diagnosed. Blood in the ventricles suggests that either the meninges or the brain parenchyma is bleeding.

3. The lumbar puncture performed during the second emergency room visit was also potentially a mistake. The rapid decrease in intracranial pressure associated with removal of cerebrospinal fluid can cause herniation of the brain downward through the tentorial notch or the foramen magnum. Such herniation can compress the respiratory center in the medulla and can rapidly lead to death. The patient's fundi should

187

CASE

remainder of the neurological and physical examination was normal. Computed tomography performed at the second hospital on the day of admission revealed subarachnoid hemorrhage. An angiogram performed on the same day revealed an aneurysm of the left posterior communicating artery (Fig. 30-1).[5] The aneurysm was surgically clipped via a left temporal craniostomy. Ventriculostomy was followed by insertion of an extraventricular drain. Initial chest radiographs were suggestive of a bibasilar pulmonary infiltrate and pulmonary edema.[6]

One week after admission, the patient's mental status deteriorated. She also had a respiratory arrest, for which she was intubated. At that time, a urine culture grew *Escherichia coli* and a sputum culture grew gram-positive coagulase-negative staphylococci. Cultures of multiple cerebral spinal fluid specimens taken over the next ten days also grew gram-positive coagulase-negative staphylococci.[7] The patient was treated intravenously with the antibiotics nafcillin and gentamicin, but her condition did not improve. The extraventricular drain was removed three weeks after admission. The patient's temperature was spiking daily. Xenon blood flow studies showed globally decreased blood flow (Fig. 30-2). By one month after admission, she was nearly comatose. Her general condition continued to deteriorate, and she died one week later.[8]

Autopsy results showed a ruptured berry aneurysm with extensive subarachnoid hemorrhage and acute and chronic inflammation of leptomeningeal vessels (Figs. 30-3 and 30-4). Despite the patient's frequent episodes of respiratory tract infection, her lungs were reasonably normal at autopsy. The cause of death was considered to be the ruptured aneurysm with subsequent complications of intracranial hemorrhage and meningitis.[9]

DISCUSSION

have been carefully evaluated for evidence of papilledema (indicating increased intracranial pressure). It would also have been helpful if the computed tomogram had been properly interpreted. Increased intracranial pressure is, unfortunately, as in this case, not always clinically suspected. If unsuspected increased pressure is found during lumbar puncture, no more cerebrospinal fluid should be removed. Instead, the cerebrospinal fluid in the manometer can be used for culture and cytology studies.

4. Administration of the potent diuretic furosemide may decrease intracranial pressure by forced diuresis. The corticosteroid dexamethasone reduces inflammation and may also consequently reduce intracranial pressure when inflammation is a significant contributing factor.

5. Lethargy and failure to recognize the place and time suggest generalized central nervous system dysfunction. Subarachnoid hemorrhage due to bleeding from a ruptured aneurysm in the circle of Willis provides an adequate explanation of the patient's symptoms and clinical findings up to the time of surgery.

6. Surgical clipping of an aneurysm prevents further hemorrhage in some patients. Insertion of a drain through the cortex to a lateral ventricle permits cerebrospinal fluid to be drawn off periodically. This reduces intracranial pressure and provides a source of cerebrospinal fluid for culture. These pulmonary findings may have been unrelated to the patient's bleeding aneurysm. Alternatively, a lethargic patient who has also been vomiting is vulnerable to developing an aspiration pneumonia.

7. The patient's respiratory arrest was probably secondary to neurological dysfunction rather than to pneumonia. Hypoxia or metabolic disturbances secondary to pneumonia may have been contributing to the neurological dysfunction. The patient's course was complicated by the development of meningitis, pneumonia, and urinary tract infections. Infection of the cerebrospinal fluid was probably introduced via the extraventricular drain.

8. Many antibiotics penetrate the blood-brain barrier only poorly, and so control of meningeal infections may be difficult. Additionally, the patient's staphylococcal infections were presumed to be hospital-acquired infections and may have been highly resistant to multiple antibiotics. Removal of the extraventricu-

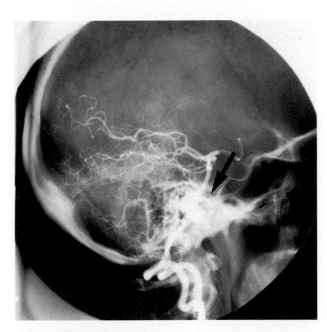

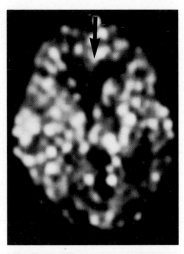

Fig. 30-2. Xenon blood flow studies show globally decreased blood flow as indicated by darkness of most areas of the brain shown in this image. This decreased blood flow probably contributed to the patient's poor neurological state. The lateral and third ventricles are visible *(arrow)*.

Fig. 30-1. Intracerebral hemorrhage from a berry aneurysm demonstrated by angiography of the vertebral system. The hemorrhage shows as a white smear *(arrow)* at the base of the skull.

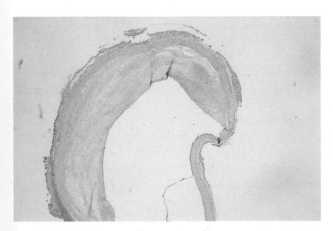

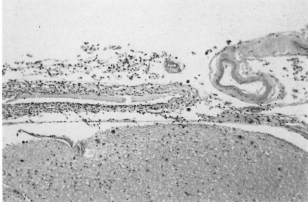

Fig. 30-3. Berry aneurysm (low power photomicrograph, hematoxylin and eosin). On the left, the arterial wall is thickened by atherosclerosis; on the right, the wall is thinned by the berry aneurysm. This thin vessel wall can rupture, producing significant intracranial hemorrhage.

Fig. 30-4. Leptomeningitis (high power photomicrograph, hematoxylin and eosin). The leptomeningeal vessels are above; the brain parenchyma is below. The leptomeningeal vessels show acute and chronic inflammation. The vein *(left)* is more affected than the artery *(right)*. High power observation of the cellular infiltrate around the vein revealed that it was composed predominantly of lymphocytes but did contain a few neutrophils.

DISCUSSION

lar drain is indicated when intracranial pressures appear to have stabilized.

9. Acute and chronic inflammation of leptomeningeal vessels reflects both the irritation produced by hemorrhage and the documented meningeal infections that had been present since at least one week after admission. The fact that the patient's lungs were reasonably normal indicates that antibiotic control of the pneumonia was more successful than was control of the meningitis, even though the same organism was involved in both processes. Lungs have a remarkable ability to recover from even severe pneumonia as long as the underlying pulmonary architecture is not damaged.

Berry Aneurysms

Aneurysms can form at the branch points of medium-sized arteries, particularly when the branch comes off at a sharp angle. There is often a defect in the wall primarily as a result of the mechanical problem of evenly wrapping two tubular structures that join together. Such aneurysms are known as *berry aneurysms* or *congenital aneurysms*. One place where such aneurysms commonly form is in the vessels in the circle of Willis at the base of the brain. This propensity may reflect the combination of relatively high flow and high pressure in the vessels and lack of adequate mechanical support for the circle of Willis. Hypertension appears to be a contributing factor in development of the aneurysmal dilation at congenitally vulnerable sites.

Berry aneurysms may remain intact and completely asymptomatic throughout life. If rupture does occur, it is often during strenuous exercise. Abrupt onset of an excruciating headache is a typical presenting symptom. Approximately half the patients become unconscious for minutes to hours. Since the vessels of the circle of Willis lie in the subarachnoid space, rupture typically produces subarachnoid hemorrhage. Such subarachnoid hemorrhage tends to compress the brain relatively evenly. Few focal or lateralizing signs may be produced,

in contrast to thromboembolic phenomena causing stroke. Increased intracranial pressure may not be present. Lumbar puncture characteristically reveals bloody cerebrospinal fluid. Nuchal rigidity, a pronounced stiffness of the neck reflecting meningeal irritation, may be present.

The rupture of an aneurysm and subsequent hemorrhage contributes to serious morbidity and mortality in several ways. The initial hemorrhage may directly destroy brain tissue, through loss of blood flow and pressure, causing stroke. The combination of external pressure and irritating fluid in the meninges can trigger arterial spasm in other intracranial vessels that may not be in the distribution of the bleeding artery. This can be particularly dangerous if atherosclerosis has narrowed the arterial lumen. Finally, berry aneurysms, unless surgically corrected, are notorious for repeatedly rebleeding, each time with increasing damage to the patient. Overall, approximately 50% of patients with rupture of a berry aneurysm die within 30 days.

Questions

1. What were this patient's presenting complaints? Where was she first seen by medical personnel?

What happened after her first emergency room visit? What happened at her second emergency room visit? Why was she transferred to a university hospital?

2. What was the patient's condition at the time of transfer to the university hospital? What studies were performed to evaluate her neurological status? What operative procedure was performed? Was the surgery successful?

3. Why was this patient vulnerable to contracting infections? Which infections did she contract? How was she treated? How did she die? What was found at autopsy?

Selected Reading

Schievink WI, Karemaker JM, Hageman LM, van der Werf DJ: Circumstances surrounding aneurysmal subarachnoid hemorrhage. Surg Neurol 32:266–272, 1989.

Stebbens WE: Etiology of intracranial berry aneurysm. J Neurosurg 70:823–831, 1989.

31 GLIOBLASTOMA MULTIFORME IN A DIABETIC PATIENT

Key Words | *meningioma, glioblastoma multiforme, breast cancer*

CASE

An elderly diabetic woman was in a fair state of health until the age of 62, when she began to have chronic headaches without mental status change or cognitive dysfunction. Six months later, a right frontotemporal meningioma was diagnosed and then excised with no complications.[1] Fifteen months after removal of the meningioma, the patient was admitted for uncontrolled diabetes. A right breast mass was discovered during this admission. Surgical removal of the mass revealed a small focus of infiltrating ductal carcinoma with no axillary masses.[2] The patient tolerated the procedure with no complications. She was discharged two weeks later with a blood glucose level fluctuating between 150 and 200 mg/100 ml (normal fasting glucose level, 75 to 110 mg/100 ml). Two months later, approximately two years after her chronic headaches started, the patient was readmitted with hyperglycemia (blood glucose level, 602 mg/100 ml) and confusion.[3]

After the blood glucose level had returned to normal limits, the patient still showed mild residual intermittent confusion. Computed tomography of the head revealed a diffuse enhancement along the medial aspect of the right temporal horn. The differential diagnosis included lymphoma, meningioma, and neoplasm of another origin. Resection of the lesion showed a second

DISCUSSION

1. Chronic headaches are associated with a wide variety of disorders. Intracranial tumor is a cause of chronic headaches that is sometimes unsuspected since more benign causes are much more common. Meningiomas are usually benign and typically have the form of a spherical mass that indents the underlying cortex.
2. Many women do not examine their own breasts on a regular basis. Consequently, the incidental identification of a breast mass is still, unfortunately, fairly common. Meningiomas are known to occur more frequently in women with breast cancer, possibly because some meningiomas contain estrogen and progesterone receptors.
3. Diabetes in elderly patients may be difficult to control for a variety of reasons, including irregular eating habits, coexisting conditions affecting memory, and infections. Elderly diabetic patients with poorly controlled diabetes who are not insulin-dependent are likely to develop profound dehydration secondary to a sustained hyperglycemic diuresis. Such patients may eventually experience hyperosmolar nonketogenic diabetic coma or may be identified at an earlier stage as a result of confusion and hyperglycemia, as was the case for this patient. Appropriate treatment usually consists of large volumes of intravenous fluids and small amounts of insulin.
4. Persistence of residual confusion together with a history of meningioma raises the question of a possible

CASE

meningioma. The patient was discharged in good stable condition two weeks after admission.[4]

Two months later, her confusion and disorientation had not improved and appeared to be slowly increasing. Repeated computed tomography of the head followed by a stereotactic biopsy showed glioblastoma multiforme of the splenium of the corpus callosum (Fig. 31-1). The patient's condition was discussed with her family. A decision was made to proceed with a course of radiation therapy. This was intended mainly to prolong her life expectancy and was not expected to markedly affect her intellectual cognitive impairment. Dexamethasone and phenytoin therapy was started.[5] The final admission occurred several months later, after the patient experienced fever and confusion. The clinical impression was that the cause of the fever was a urinary tract infection, since culture of a urine specimen grew *Proteus mirabilis*. The fever disappeared after antibiotic therapy with ampicillin and gentamicin. The patient was discharged to a nursing home ten days after admission.[6] During the two weeks following discharge, she again developed fever and became progressively obtunded. She developed periodic breathing for a few days and then died in her sleep.[7]

An autopsy performed on the patient's embalmed body showed occlusion of the right pulmonary artery by recent thromboembolus. Extensive patchy bronchopneumonia was present in both lungs (Fig. 31-2). Aspirated vegetable particles and clusters of fungal yeast forms were observed.[8] Examination of the brain revealed a glioblastoma multiforme (Figs. 31-3 and 31-4). The tumor involved deep white matter, occipital and posterior parietal lobes, posterior fornices, the splenium of the corpus callosum, and the right hippocampal formation. Changes of post-radiation encephalopathy were noted. There was ventriculomegaly of all ventricles. There was minimal cerebrovascular atherosclerosis. Portions of dura mater obtained at autopsy from the right middle fossa revealed residual meningioma.[9] The kidneys showed arteriosclerosis and arteriolosclerosis with bilateral acute papillary necrosis and bacterial clumps. There was no evidence of residual

DISCUSSION

recurrence of the tumor. This led to the identification of a second meningioma, which was then removed.

5. The resection was expected to either improve or stabilize the patient's condition. When the symptoms continued to progress, the search for an explanation was reinitiated. The stereotactic biopsy identified the presence of a previously unrecognized tumor, glioblastoma multiforme. Glioblastoma multiforme is an aggressive tumor derived from the astrocyte cell line. The prognosis is very poor. Radiation therapy will prolong life from an expectancy of about four months to approximately one year. Corticosteroids such as dexamethasone reduce cerebral edema and can consequently often lower intracranial pressure and improve cerebral function. Patients with intracranial tumors often develop epilepsy, and the phenytoin was administered prophylactically to prevent this complication.

6. *Proteus mirabilis* is an aggressive organism that can cause serious ascending urinary tract infections. Diabetic patients are particularly vulnerable to urinary tract infection, probably because of immunosuppression. Glucose in the urine of diabetic patients with poorly controlled diabetes may also provide a rich medium that enhances bacterial growth. Immunosuppression secondary to steroid therapy may have also increased the patient's vulnerability to both urinary tract infection and the bronchopneumonia found at autopsy.

7. *Periodic breathing* is breathing interrupted by long pauses. Increasing cognitive impairment and periodic breathing suggest brainstem damage, possibly by tumor or edema.

8. A patient in a nursing home may be embalmed before a physician looks at the final clinical record. In such cases, if an autopsy appears appropriate, it can still be performed on the embalmed body. Some tissue damage occurs during the delay and the embalming process, and consequently the microscopic findings may be more difficult to interpret than in a normal autopsy. Unsuspected findings at autopsy included thromboembolus in the right pulmonary artery and extensive pneumonia in both lungs. Pulmonary embolism often occurs in bedridden patients. Patients with seriously depressed consciousness are often unable to cooperate during feeding and are

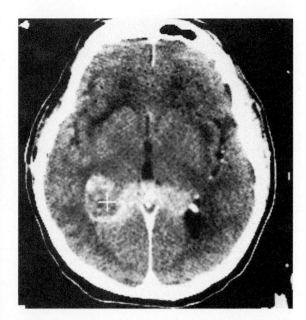

Fig. 31-1. Glioblastoma multiforme. A large tumor mass *(white)* has spread via the corpus callosum to involve both cerebral hemispheres. An area of possible tumor necrosis is indicated *(cross)*.

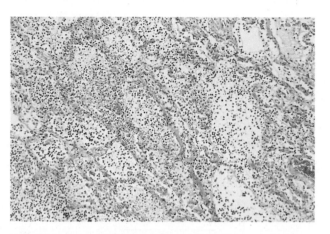

Fig. 31-2. Pneumonia (low power photomicrograph, hematoxylin and eosin). Bilateral bronchopneumonia, with intra-alveolar hemorrhage, inflammatory cells, and cellular debris, contributed to this patient's death. The pneumonia was probably a result of aspiration since vegetable particles and clusters of yeasts (not shown) were found in some bronchi.

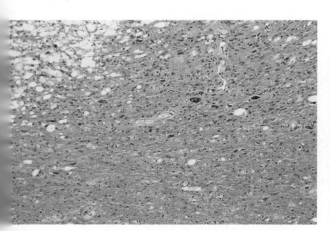

Fig. 31-3. Glioblastoma multiforme (low power photomicrograph, hematoxylin and eosin). Brain parenchyma is in the lower right; tumor is in the upper left. The tumor margin is not easily recognizable.

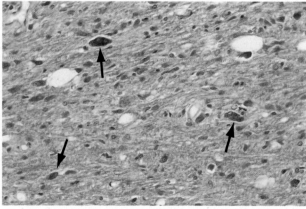

Fig. 31-4. Glioblastoma multiforme (high power photomicrograph, hematoxylin and eosin). This high power field taken from the tumor margin shows isolated large, bizarre nuclei *(arrows)* present between otherwise relatively normal brain parenchymal cells. This tumor is very difficult to treat in part because its boundaries are poorly defined and isolated tumor cells can be found deep within the adjacent brain.

CASE

breast carcinoma or any metastatic breast tumor. The cause of death was probably a combination of recent pulmonary embolism and bilateral bronchopneumonia, with urinary tract infection as a contributing factor, in a patient with glioblastoma multiforme.[10]

DISCUSSION

consequently vulnerable to aspiration. Such aspiration may be demonstrated at autopsy by the finding of aspirated vegetable particles within the lungs.

9. Glioblastoma multiforme is a very invasive tumor that tends to occur predominantly in white matter. It often crosses from one cerebral hemisphere to the other via the corpus callosum. Neurons are relatively resistant to direct radiation damage because they do not divide. However, radiation can damage both blood vessels, potentially causing parenchymal necrosis, and astrocytes, causing a reactive gliosis. Ventriculomegaly can occur either as a result of impairment in the circulation of cerebrospinal fluid (perhaps due to partial obstruction by tumor) or secondary to loss of tissue during radiation therapy.

10. Acute papillary necrosis occurs in some severe upper urinary tract infections. Arteriosclerotic and arteriolosclerotic changes are probably the result of hypertension and diabetes.

Brain Tumors

Tumors in the central nervous system can arise either through metastasis from systemic cancer or as primary tumors. Either class of tumor can produce neurological impairment by compression or infiltration of the brain. The specific neurological findings usually reflect the location and rate of growth of the tumor more strongly than they reflect the type of tumor. Headache, progressive generalized decline in cognitive ability, and focal neurological signs are common presenting complaints. Increased intracranial pressure can impair retinal venous return and produce papilledema. Expanding cranial masses can produce a variety of herniation syndromes characterized by specific focal signs coupled with depression of consciousness. Defects in mentation, language, or movement may help to localize the tumor mass.

Tumors derived from the astrocyte line range from well-differentiated to anaplastic, and their effect correspondingly ranges from relatively benign to capable of producing death in less than 18 months. Glioblastoma multiforme is the most common, anaplastic, and dangerous of the astrocyte neoplasms. It is characteristically very invasive, will frequently cross the corpus callosum, and often outgrows its blood supply. Cancerous transformation of oligodendroglia produces a usually slowly growing oligodendroglioma. It is characteristically located in the frontal lobes or within the ventricles of mature adults. Tumors derived from cells of the pia-arachnoid are termed *meningiomas* and may be either benign or malignant. They usually occur on the external surface of the brain, particularly along the midline. Meningiomas typically produce a well-defined nodule that compresses the underlying brain without invading it. Ependymomas are typically located within the ventricular system and may impede the circulation of cerebrospinal fluid. Primitive neuroectodermal cells can differentiate into neurons, glia, and skeletal muscle. They are the most primitive cell line capable of producing primary brain tumors. Medulloblastoma is the most common variety of these primitive neuroectodermal tumors. It accounts for one-quarter of brain tumors in children and also occurs in young adults. Medulloblastomas are typically located in the midline, often in the cerebellar vermis, and are composed of small, densely staining cells. A similar tumor, neuroblastoma, also occurs in the cells derived from neural crest in the adrenal medulla. Finally, a variety of other tumors are derived from other cells in the cranium. These include lymphomas, craniopharyngiomas derived from Rathke's pouch, pinealomas, pituitary adenomas, dermoid cysts, lipomas, and hemangioblastomas.

Questions

1. This patient's history is notable for the several tumors that she developed. Which of her tumors were benign? Malignant? How was each tumor diagnosed and treated? Which treatments were successful?
2. What symptoms can brain tumors cause? What neurological symptoms did this patient initially experience? How did her neurological symptoms change with time? Interpreting the clinical history in retrospect, what do you think were the relative roles of her two meningiomas and her glioblastoma multiforme?
3. Describe this patient's terminal course. What role did infection play? What was found at autopsy?

Selected Reading

Baumann CK, Zumwalt CB: Intracranial neoplasms. An overview. AORN J 50:240, 242, 244–248, 1989.

Knuckley NW, Stoll J Jr, Epstein MH: Intracranial and spinal meningiomas in patients with breast carcinoma: case reports. Neurosurgery 25:112–116, 1989.

32 ACOUSTIC NERVE SHEATH TUMOR COMPLICATED BY CEREBRAL HEMORRHAGE

Key Words | nerve sheath tumor, cerebral hemorrhage, surgical complications

CASE

The patient was a 58-year-old woman with a four-year history of left-sided diminished hearing associated with vertigo, gait unsteadiness, occipital headaches, and a tendency to fall to the left.[1] Three years before admission, computed tomography was performed and was reported to show no evidence of tumor.[2] She was treated with the antiemetic meclizine, but her symptoms gradually worsened.[3] She was admitted two months before her death, complaining of palpitations and headaches. The evaluation of her headache included computed tomography, which revealed a 4.5-cm mass in the left cerebellar pontine angle.[4] Mitral valve prolapse with associated paroxysmal atrial fibrillation was identified during the same admission (Fig. 32-1).[5]

The patient was readmitted two months later for resection of the tumor.[6] Her physical status was good. Neurological findings on the right were normal. Neurological findings on the left consisted of absent hearing, diminished nasal labial fold, diminished sensation to pinprick in the sec-

DISCUSSION

1. The combination of diminished hearing and symptoms attributable to vestibular dysfunction strongly suggests that either the inner ear or the acoustic nerve was impaired.
2. Computed tomography performed to identify possible tumor involvement was originally negative and several years later became positive for a mass. This indicates one of the limitations of computed tomography: a lesion may be too small to be adequately visualized by the scan but can still, if located in a critical area, be sufficiently large to be symptomatic.
3. Meclizine is an antihistamine with antiemetic activity that is particularly useful when vertigo, nausea, and vomiting are secondary to vestibular disease.
4. Headache in the presence of known neurological deficits again raised the possibility of intracranial tumor. Palpitations (perceptions of a rapid and intense beating of the heart) were an unrelated symptom probably attributable to the paroxysmal atrial fibrillation demonstrated during the same admission. This illustrates a fundamental point sometimes missed by beginning physicians: although it is tempt-

CASE

ond and third divisions of the trigeminal nerve, and diminished corneal reflex. The impression was left acoustic nerve sheath tumor with evidence of seventh and fifth cranial nerve compression.[7]

Three days after admission the patient underwent a craniotomy with resection of the left acoustic nerve sheath tumor (Fig. 32-2). The operation was complicated by excessive bleeding, and removal of the entire tumor was not possible.[8] Postoperatively, the bleeding persisted and computed tomography revealed a cerebellar hematoma. The patient was returned to surgery for evacuation of this clot.[9] She remained in a persistent coma postoperatively, and repeated tomography revealed necrosis of the remaining tumor with swelling of the brain. She was returned to the operating room for revision of the excision and evaluation of the left cerebellar clot.[10] Postoperatively she had no cranial nerve reflexes and no response to deep pain. Tomography revealed massive hemorrhage involving the midbrain, thalamus, and cerebellum with intraventricular blood and hydrocephalus.[11] Her condition progressively deteriorated, and she was pronounced dead. Permission for an autopsy of the head only was obtained.[12]

Autopsy of the head confirmed the presence of serious hemorrhage: a 250-ml subdural hematoma was present in the left posterior fossa and intraventricular hemorrhage was also present. A fragment of necrotic tissue resembling the original tumor was found in the left cerebellar pontine angle. The left lateral brainstem was infarcted and demonstrated foci of recent hemorrhage in the midbrain and upper pons (Fig. 32-3). Herniation of the cerebellar tonsils had also occurred.[13]

DISCUSSION

ing to search for a single explanation for all findings, sometimes two independent processes occur concurrently.

5. Mitral valve prolapse is a clinical syndrome with a variety of causes, in which excessive tissue in the mitral valve produces abnormal valve function that can be detected by auscultation as a clicking sound. In most patients, mitral valve prolapse is a benign and asymptomatic condition. In those few patients with more serious disease, involvement of the conduction system adjacent to the valve may produce arrhythmias, which may in turn produce palpitations, lightheadedness, syncope, and, very rarely, sudden death. Infective endocarditis, thrombus formation, or both, may also involve the affected leaflets and be a source of cerebral emboli.

6. Given the slow progression of the patient's symptoms over several years, it was feasible to schedule the surgery electively.

7. Nerve sheath tumors, also known as neurilemmomas, are benign tumors of Schwann cells. The tentative diagnosis of acoustic nerve sheath tumor was made because of the characteristic location of the tumor coupled with its localized neurological signs and absence of any indication of metastasis. A 4.5-cm mass is relatively large considering the confined space of the cranium. It is consequently not surprising that headaches were present and that the tumor had apparently involved the adjacent facial and trigeminal cranial nerves to produce diminished labial fold, diminished sensation to pinprick, and diminished corneal reflex.

8. This was a large tumor and required a substantial blood supply. Such tumors may bleed easily, as apparently happened in this patient.

9. Hemorrhage after cranial surgery is particularly dangerous because in the confined space of the cranium, even a relatively small volume of blood, tumor, or edema may be sufficient to produce compression of and damage to vital brainstem structures. Surgical evacuation of the clot was consequently important therapeutically.

10. Unfortunately, the patient had entered a coma with demonstrated edema of the brain, from which it was not possible to arouse her.

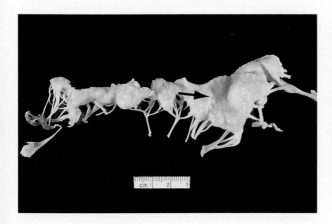

Fig. 32-1. Mitral valve prolapse (gross specimen, from another case). This mitral valve was removed at surgery. Portions of the valve are thinned and increased in width *(arrow)*. These changes are characteristic of mitral valve prolapse.

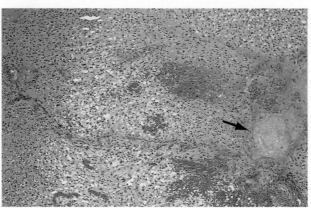

Fig. 32-2. Acoustic neuroma (low power photomicrograph, hematoxylin and eosin). This benign tumor fills the entire field. The tumor tends to form two distinct histological patterns. Densely packed spindle cells *(left)* are known as Antoni A tissue; loosely packed pleomorphic cells with prominent pale cytoplasm *(center)* are known as Antoni B tissue. Despite the different appearances, these two tissues are derived from immunologically similar tumor cells. An area of tumor necrosis surrounded by hemorrhage is present *(arrow)*.

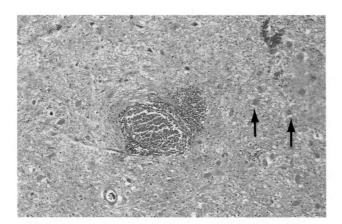

Fig. 32-3. Hemorrhage within the brainstem (high power photomicrograph, hematoxylin and eosin). In the center of the field there is a focus of hemorrhage around a small vein in the brainstem parenchyma. Nearby neuron nuclei *(arrows)* appear smudged, suggesting neuronal cell death. The smaller glial nuclei are relatively preserved. Infarction with hemorrhage in the patient's left lateral brainstem probably contributed to her poor postoperative neurological state.

DISCUSSION

11. The combination of absence of cranial reflexes and no response to deep pain is presumptive evidence of death of much of the brainstem. This clinical diagnosis was substantiated by the evidence of massive intracranial hemorrhage.

12. This patient's history illustrates a common therapeutic dilemma to which there is often no clear answer: repeated surgery may be necessary to correct conditions that are immediately life-threatening, but it always carries the risk of exacerbating rather than alleviating the patient's problems. In general, surgeons attempt to stabilize a seriously ill patient as much as possible before even emergency surgery, even if only to delay surgery for an hour or so to partially correct an electrolyte imbalance. Such correction is not always possible when the patient's condition is immediately life-threatening.

13. The infarction of the brainstem demonstrated at autopsy was probably the result of compression of vessels by the mass of hemorrhage at the surgical site. Brainstem infarction explains the patient's severe neurological findings of coma accompanied by absence of cranial reflexes and response to pain. When either such infarction or milder ischemic damage occurs, it tends to exacerbate the problems with brainstem compression since the damaged tissue tends to swell with edema. The cerebellar tonsils are one of several sites in the brain that are particularly vulnerable for anatomical reasons to damage and herniation in the presence of increased intracranial pressure. The cingulate gyrus and the anterior portion of the hippocampus are also particularly vulnerable to herniation.

Nerve Sheath Tumors

Benign tumors of Schwann cells can arise wherever Schwann cells myelinate nerves, and thus they occur in cranial and spinal nerve roots as well as in peripheral nerve trunks. Historically, these tumors have been divided into classes depending upon whether they occur predominantly within or adjacent to the nerve. Multiple tumors within the nerve, known as neurofibromas, are typically associated with a hereditary condition known as von Recklinghausen's disease or neurofibromatosis. Tumors adjacent to the nerve more commonly occur singly and have a variety of names including neurilemmomas, schwannomas, and nerve sheath tumors. Although this classification has been, and still is, widely used, the validity of the distinction has been challenged by some investigators since careful examination of a nerve sheath tumor may show tumor within the nerve and careful examination of a neurofibroma may show regions of tumor in which no apparent nerve is present.

Symptoms produced by a nerve sheath tumor are usually related either to dysfunction of the involved nerve or to compression of adjacent structures. The cranial nerve most frequently involved with a nerve sheath tumor is the eighth, or acoustic, nerve. This nerve passes next to the cerebellopontine angle in its course from the inner ear to the brainstem; consequently, an acoustic nerve sheath tumor may present as a mass in the cerebellopontine angle. When the tumor becomes sufficiently large, adjacent cranial nerves become involved in a typical order. Unilateral hearing loss and vestibular dysfunction occur first and indicate involvement of the original acoustic nerve. Later, the increasing volume of the tumor stretches the ipsilateral facial nerve and then the trigeminal nerve, producing first sensory and then motor dysfunction on the face. Eventually, cerebellar and brainstem compression occurs.

Questions

1. What symptoms did this patient initially experience?

Each of the patient's symptoms, taken singly, is nonspecific and has multiple relatively benign causes. Which combinations of symptoms would you consider sufficiently disturbing to want to proceed with an extensive evaluation of the patient? How was she evaluated?

2. What types of processes can cause masses in the head? What is a neurilemmoma? Which structures might a relatively large mass in the cerebellar pontine angle directly or indirectly affect? What symptoms would be produced? Which of these symptoms did this patient experience?

3. What are the risks of brain surgery? For which of these risks was the patient particularly vulnerable? What happened to her intraoperatively and then postoperatively? Discuss the relationship of the autopsy findings to the patient's clinical course.

Selected Reading

Ariel IM: Tumors of the peripheral nervous system. Semin Surg Oncol 4:7–12, 1988.

Gorman WF: Early diagnosis of acoustic neuroma. J Okla State Med Assoc 81:283–287, 1988.

ENDOCRINE ORGANS

33 CARCINOMA OF THE BREAST

Key Words | breast cancer, metastatic disease, pneumonia

CASE

The patient had been found to have breast cancer eight years previously, at age 57, when biopsy of a lump in her right breast showed adenocarcinoma. The right breast was removed by radical mastectomy, and she was treated with chemotherapy.[1] Five years later, cancerous nodules were found in the remaining breast, which was also removed by radical mastectomy. The patient had been treated with radiotherapy for a metastatic lesion in the right femur and then later with internal fixation for pathological fracture of the same bone.[2]

Over the six months preceding admission, the patient received radiation therapy for pain due to metastases in her legs, lumbosacral spine, ribs, and one elbow. A myelogram performed two months before admission showed extradural L4-5 compression secondary to a herniated disk (Fig. 33-1).[3] During the one and one-half months preceding admission, she was given a course of chemotherapy that included fluorouracil, methotrexate, and cyclophosphamide. She was then admitted because of failure to thrive and increasing difficulty in walking. Four days before admission, her daughter noticed that for the first time the patient had become incontinent of stool and urine.[4]

Her physical examination was notable principally for marked proximal muscular weakness of both legs, moderate peripheral edema, and scattered basilar rales in the lungs. A chest radiograph

DISCUSSION

1. Lumps in breasts can be due to many different causes including breast cancer, cystic disease, fat necrosis, and adenofibromas. Biopsy is considered to be the definitive diagnostic procedure and should be performed promptly since many breast cancers metastasize early. In radical mastectomy, the breast is removed together with the underlying pectoral muscles and the axillary lymph nodes. Radical mastectomies are no longer commonly performed because survival rates after less disfiguring surgery appear comparable.

2. Women who have had cancer in one breast are at increased risk of developing cancer in the other breast. The presence of cancer in the remaining breast may indicate either the presence of new cancer or recurrence of the original cancer. The lesion in the femur is evidence that the cancer was metastasizing widely. In these circumstances, surgical therapy usually is not useful. Therapeutic options included chemotherapy, which had been previously unsuccessful, and palliative radiation therapy. Radiation therapy was chosen and was repeated later many times in many different regions of the patient's body. When it became clear that the radiation therapy was failing to control the cancer, another course of chemotherapy was chosen.

3. Breast cancer has a propensity for metastasizing to bone. Invasion of the cancer into bone will cause lytic lesions that can be very painful. These lesions are also vulnerable to pathological fractures in response to stress as minimal as that caused by standing. Pathological fractures can produce collapse of vertebrae. Such

CASE

showed opacification of the left mid-lung field, with a suggestion of volume loss and atelectasis. Extensive lytic disease of the left shoulder was also present. A radiograph of the lumbosacral region showed severe degeneration and lytic disease of the lumbosacral spine and sacrum, with a new collapse of lumbar vertebra L-1. Computed tomography of the brain demonstrated bony destruction of the left occipital condyle consistent with metastatic deposits. Serum calcium levels were within normal limits.[5]

The patient was lethargic. There was further progression of her paresis. She developed fever and an elevated leukocyte count one week after admission. Culture of a urine specimen grew *Cryptococcus neoformans*, which was the only apparent possible source of infection. On the same day, 600 ml of pink-yellow fluid was aspirated by thoracocentesis from the left pleural cavity. Results of a cytological examination of this specimen were negative.[6] The patient remained very lethargic. Culture of a cerebrospinal fluid specimen obtained ten days after admission grew the same strain of *C. neoformans* as had been isolated in the urine. Five days later, the patient complained of left leg pain. Her legs were cold, and her pulses were diminished. Vascular surgery consultation was obtained. The impression was that the pain could not be explained by arterial insufficiency in light of the clinical examination and the Doppler ultrasonography. The clinical impression at that time was that the pain was of neurogenic origin.[7]

The patient complained of dyspnea three weeks after admission. The periods of dyspnea increased, and she died two days later. The autopsy demonstrated widespread metastasis to the lungs, hilar lymph nodes, paratracheal lymph nodes, bone, liver, and both adrenal glands (Figs. 33-2 and 33-3). Evidence of cryptococcal infection was also present in the meninges and central nervous system parenchyma (Fig. 33-4). A marked granulomatous reaction accompanied the leptomeningitis and indicated that the process had been continuing for some time and was therefore subacute in evolution. There was evidence of both cryptococcal and staphylococcal pneumo-

DISCUSSION

vertebral collapse can lead to herniated disks, pain due to the compression of spinal cord and nerve roots, and eventually loss of functions carried by the ventral roots.

4. Difficulty in walking and urinary incontinence suggest that the lumbosacral nerve roots either have been infiltrated with cancer or are being compressed by collapsing vertebrae. "Failure to thrive" refers to poorly defined signs and symptoms of illness such as fatigue, loss of appetite, and failure to gain weight despite attempts to do so. Although this sign is nonspecific, it is clinically significant and suggests serious underlying disease. In this patient, it suggests that the patient's tumor burden has reached the point of impairing her body's ability to meet physiological needs.

5. Proximal muscle weakness suggests damage to peripheral nerves. Such damage may be due to metastases involving nerves, nerve root compression related to pathological vertebral fractures, or radiation damage. In the absence of cardiac abnormalities, peripheral edema may have been due to impairment of lymphatic drainage by tumor involvement of the legs. The presence of scattered basilar rales suggests possible pneumonia. Tumor occlusion of smaller bronchi and bronchioles can cause atelectasis of distal alveoli as the entrapped gas is slowly resorbed by the body. These lesions indicate increasingly extensive tumor metastasis to bone. Serum calcium levels are often elevated in patients with extensive bone metastases.

6. This patient's lethargy has several possible causes, including tumor involvement of the brain, toxicity of chemotherapeutic agents, meningitis, and metabolic disturbances. The word *paresis* refers to the patient's proximal muscular weakness. The presence of fever and an elevated leukocyte count suggests infection. Cancer involving the lung and pleura can produce pleural effusion. Alternatively, the pleural effusion may have been due to pleural involvement by adjacent pneumonia or abscess. *C. neoformans* is a yeastlike fungus that acts as an opportunistic pathogen primarily in immunosuppressed hosts.

7. Isolation of *Cryptococcus* from spinal fluid indicates that meningitis may be contributing to the patient's neurological state. Possible vascular insufficiency might have been due to either atherosclerosis or tumor involvement of the vessels. Doppler ultrasonography can noninvasively quantify blood flow

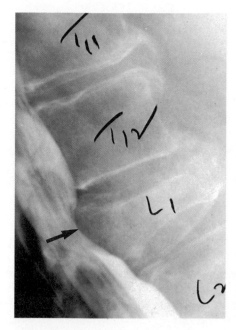

Fig. 33-1. Vertebral compression secondary to breast cancer metastasis. The myelogram shows compression of L-1 vertebrae with protrusion *(arrow)* into the spinal canal.

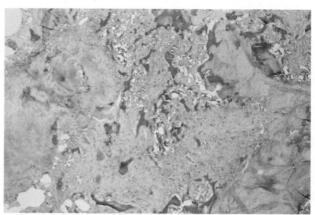

Fig. 33-2. Breast cancer involving bone marrow (low power photomicrograph, hematoxylin and eosin). The normal bone marrow has been almost completely replaced by masses of tumor.

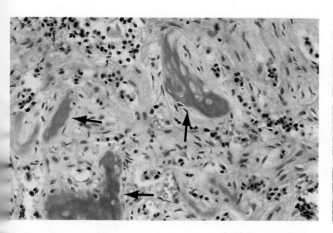

Fig. 33-3. Breast cancer involving bone marrow, detail of Fig. 33-2 (high power photomicrograph, hematoxylin and eosin). This micrograph shows that the tumor is destroying the normal bone spicules *(arrows)*. Neovascularization is visible as multiple small vessels containing erythrocytes. Many of the tumor cells resemble fibrous tissue.

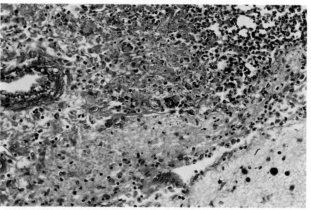

Fig. 33-4. Cryptococcal meningitis (high power photomicrograph, mucicarmine, from another case). The capsules of the yeast form of *Cryptococcus* are visible as small red ovals approximately the size of nuclei *(upper right)*. The larger red structures in the brain cortex *(lower right)* are corpora amylacea, commonly found in older brains. The cryptococcal infection has caused perivascular hemorrhage and a cellular proliferation in the meninges.

CASE

nia. The cause of death was considered to be wide-spread metastatic disease and pneumonia complicating breast carcinoma.[8]

DISCUSSION

through superficial vessels. The fact that Doppler studies did not confirm the initial impression of vascular insufficiency illustrates that clinical impressions should be substantiated, if possible, by more objective studies.

8. It is probable both clinically and from the autopsy evidence that the patient was infected at a subacute level before her admission. Her cryptococcal meningitis probably preceded the cryptococcal and staphylococcal pneumonia since respiratory symptoms were not noted until shortly before death.

Breast Cancer

Approximately 10% of women in the United States will eventually develop adenocarcinoma of the breast. Breast cancer is a disease mainly of older women, with median age at diagnosis of about 60 years. A family history of breast cancer is one of only a few recognized risk factors, but 90% of patients with breast cancer do not have female relatives with a history of the disease. Most diagnoses are made by finding a mass during breast self-examination. Current American Cancer Society guidelines suggest that a baseline mammogram should be performed at age 35. Routine mammograms should then be subsequently performed every other year from age 40 to 49, and yearly thereafter.

Many different histological types of adenocarcinoma of the breast occur, including infiltrating ductal, medullary, mucinous, tubular, and papillary carcinoma. The specific histological type of cancer is usually not of particular clinical interest because the therapy and prognosis of different histological types are similar. The prognosis is most accurately predicted by accurate staging of the extent of the tumor.

A small nodule found at diagnosis may have taken eight or more years to form. Therefore, it is probable that metastases have already occurred at the time of diagnosis. Chemotherapy, radiation therapy, or both, are consequently commonly used as adjunctive therapy after surgery. Although curative treatment is attempted when the tumor has no distant metastases, only palliative treatment is feasible for patients with extensive disease. Radiation therapy of local lesions may reduce pain and disability. Up to 60% of breast cancers contain re-

ceptors for estrogen, progesterone, or both, and may respond to hormonal therapy with agents such as the antiestrogen tamoxifen. Malignant pleural effusion is common and can be controlled either by closed-tube drainage of the chest or by injection of a sclerosing agent such as tetracycline into the pleural space.

Questions

1. Describe this patient's clinical course up to the time of her final admission. How had her breast cancer been treated? What was the rationale for each therapy? What are the advantages and disadvantages of the various modes of therapy for breast cancer? How successful was this patient's therapy?

2. What were the patient's presenting complaints at her final admission? What did physical examination and laboratory studies show? Describe the relationship of these findings to the patient's metastatic disease.

3. What infection(s) did the patient develop? What type of organism is *Cryptococcus*? From what sources was the organism isolated? What other problems did the patient experience? How did she die? What did the autopsy show?

Selected Reading

Spratt JS, Greenberg RA, Kuhns JG, Amin EA: Breast cancer risk: a review of definitions and assessments of risk. J Surg Oncol 41:42–46, 1989.

Townsend CM: Management of breast cancer: surgery and adjuvant therapy. Clin Symp 39(4):1–32, 1988.

34 SEPTIC ARTHRITIS IN A DIABETIC PATIENT

Key Words | diabetes, septic arthritis, amputation

CASE

The patient was a 52-year-old woman, with a history of hypertension and diabetes mellitus, who presented with a chief complaint of right knee pain with generalized weakness and malaise. The patient had fallen on her right knee 11 months previously and had had intermittent pain since that time. Approximately three weeks before admission, she again fell on her right knee and was then unable to walk.[1] The knee pain persisted. She had a decreased range of motion, and the knee joint was swollen and firm. She noted drainage from the medial surface of the knee approximately two days before admission, and over the following two days she had an increase in general malaise, anorexia, nausea, and vomiting. She denied chest pain, shortness of breath, polyuria, polydipsia, coughing and dysuria.[2]

A diagnosis of diabetes mellitus had been made five years previously, and insulin therapy was started. However, the patient had refused to take any insulin for the last one to two years. Physical examination revealed a hypotensive, obese woman with a huge effusion of the right knee with erythema, tenderness, and purulent skin ulcerations. Her mental status was poor, with intermittent lethargy and unresponsiveness.[3] Pertinent laboratory data included a normal white cell count of which 75% were immature neutrophils (normal, <5%). There was a marked elevation of serum glucose levels, and serum ketones were present. There was also elevation of blood urea nitrogen and serum creatinine.[4] An aspirate of the

DISCUSSION

1. Possible explanations for pain near a joint after injury include damage to muscles, tendons, bone, or the joint proper. Generalized weakness and malaise suggest a systemic process that may or may not be related to the joint dysfunction and pain. Some patients with serious, chronic disease do not consult a physician until very late, when it may be difficult to prevent serious morbidity or even death.

2. A swollen and firm joint with decreased range of motion suggests serious inflammation and possibly infection. Drainage from the medial surface of the knee suggests an abscess that had broken through to the surface. Steadily increasing systemic symptoms raised the possibility that the patient's probable joint infection had been complicated by bacteremia and sepsis. Questions about chest pain, shortness of breath, and cough will screen for pulmonary and cardiovascular problems such as pneumonia or myocardial infarction. Questions about polyuria and polydipsia will screen for exacerbation of diabetic symptoms. The question about dysuria was a screening question for symptoms possibly related to urinary tract infection, since a diabetic would be very prone to these infections and they might also have caused the sepsis.

3. Patients with poorly controlled diabetes are at increased risk of developing severe infections. Hypotension suggests that cardiovascular decompensation had occurred. Possible causes included myocardial infarction, congestive heart failure, hemorrhage, and sepsis. Sepsis was the most probable cause in this patient, who demonstrated clear evidence of infection

211

CASE

knee revealed numerous white and red blood cells and gram-positive cocci in clusters. Cultures of wound and blood specimens grew *Staphylococcus aureus*. Radiographs of the right lower extremity revealed erosion of the proximal right tibia with subcutaneous air.[5] The clinical impression was acute osteomyelitis and septic arthritis of the right knee. The plan for the patient's management included fluid maintenance, pressor agents, insulin, and antibiotics. It was also decided that amputation of the leg above the knee was the best course (Fig. 34-2).[6]

The hospital course following the amputation was complicated by development of oliguric acute tubular necrosis requiring dialysis; disseminated intravascular coagulation with gastrointestinal bleeding; and hemoptysis. A pericardial rub was

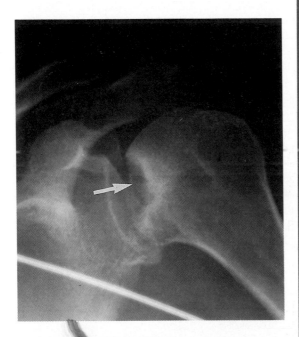

Fig. 34-1. Radiograph of the left shoulder shows a large erosion involving the medial aspect of the left humeral head adjacent to the gleno-humeral joint (arrow). This lesion is bounded by an increased bone density, indicating that the lesion is chronic. The radiological differential diagnosis included chronic osteomyelitis and localized avascular necrosis.

DISCUSSION

(see item 7 below). Neurological symptoms such as lethargy suggest that serious metabolic derangement was occurring.

4. The relatively low leukocyte count dominated by immature neutrophils suggests that marrow production of neutrophils was inadequate to control the patient's infection. Diabetic control often worsens during infection. The patient's lethargy and unresponsiveness may have been due in part to developing ketogenic diabetic coma. Elevation of blood urea nitrogen and serum creatinine levels indicates renal dysfunction, possibly as a result of diabetic glomerular disease, pyelonephritis, or renal tubular disease resulting from shock.

5. The results of aspiration of the knee were consistent with an abscess. Gram-positive cocci in clusters were probably *Staphylococcus*. Erosion of the lower tibia indicated that the infection had involved the bone. The subcutaneous air was probably introduced through the fistula through which the abscess was draining through the skin.

6. Amputation of the limb potentially controlled the infection and limited the metabolic load due to debris from the abscess.

7. The hypotension associated with sepsis can impair perfusion, leading to acute tubular necrosis and deteriorating renal function. Disseminated intravascular coagulation can occur during sepsis and may be associated with bleeding, as well as thrombus formation, because of consumption of platelets and coagulation factors. Uremia is a relatively common cause of pericarditis. The patient's episode of hemoptysis may have been related to her disseminated intravascular coagulation. Alternatively, she may have developed a bronchitis or pneumonia in addition to her other problems. Results of the bone scan suggest that osteomyelitis may also have been occurring in the scapula and pelvis.

8. Possible causes of cardiopulmonary arrest in this patient include myocardial infarction, arrhythmias, and pulmonary embolism.

9. The glomerular and renal vasculature changes are typical of longstanding diabetic renal disease. Pyelonephritis refers to infection of the kidney. Necrotizing papillitis is a severe form of pyelonephritis in which the renal papillae become necrotic. The in-

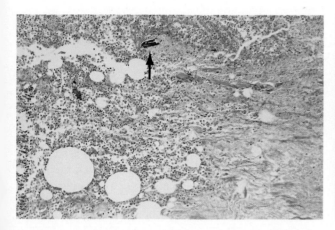

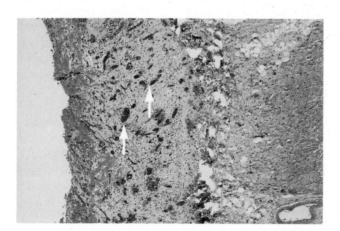

Fig. 34-2. Osteomyelitis (low power photomicrograph, hematoxylin and eosin). The normal bone marrow has been almost completely disrupted by the infection. The only remaining evidence of bone is a small fragment of necrotic bone *(arrow)*. Some marrow fat cells are still recognizable as unstained circular areas. Fibrosis has completely replaced marrow on the right.

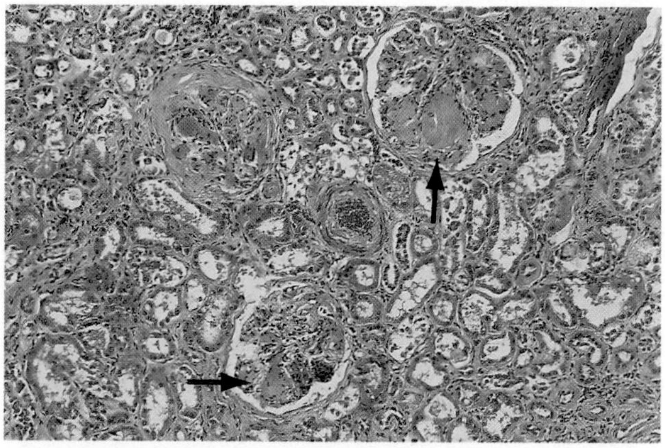

Fig. 34-3. Diabetic kidney (high power photomicrograph, hematoxylin and eosin). Three glomeruli exhibit varying stages of sclerosis. Nodular sclerosis *(arrows)* in diabetic kidneys is known as Kimmelsteil-Wilson sclerosis.

Fig. 34-4. Fibrinous pericarditis with excessive granulation tissue (low power photomicrograph, hematoxylin and eosin). The pericardium *(left)* is markedly thickened and has been replaced by granulation tissue in which prominent neovascularization *(arrows)* is present. Some hemorrhage and fibrin are seen at the pericardial surface. The muscle *(right)* is relatively unaffected.

CASE

heard that was thought to be secondary to uremia. A radiograph of the left shoulder demonstrated a large erosion of the left humeral head (Fig. 34-1). A bone scan revealed increased uptake in the left shoulder and scapula and right pelvis.[7] The patient remained stable, and her condition appeared to be improving. Unfortunately, approximately one month after admission, she was suddenly found hypotensive and apneic and could not be resuscitated.[8]

At autopsy, a variety of renal changes were observed that were considered to be related to the patient's diabetes (Fig. 34-3). The glomeruli revealed both diffuse and nodular (Kimmelstiel-Wilson) glomerulosclerosis, thickened renal tubular basement membranes, and patchy interstitial fibrosis as well as a multifocal, chronic inflammatory interstitial infiltrate. Marked hyaline arteriolonephrosclerosis was also seen, as was intimal proliferation within the interlobular arteries. Focal acute necrotizing papillitis and foci of acute pyelonephritis were also present. The wall of the genitourinary tract was diffusely thickened, and the mucosal surface was roughened and dull. Chronic inflammatory changes were observed microscopically.[9]

The left ventricle was hypertrophic, and the heart was enlarged. Both fibrinous and fibrous pericarditis were present (Fig. 34-4). Atherosclerotic disease involved the larger arteries. Hyaline arteriosclerosis was noted in microscopic sections of the spleen and ovary. Cultures of blood, spleen, and lung specimens were sterile. Cardiorespiratory arrest was considered to be the cause of death.[10]

DISCUSSION

flammatory changes observed in the bladder suggest that an ascending intraluminal infection was the cause of this patient's pyelonephritis. Her upper urinary tract infection was clinically unsuspected. Her acute tubular necrosis had resolved by the time of her death.

10. The pericarditis had been clinically suspected. The finding of fibrin deposits on the pericardium suggested that the pericarditis was a continuing process. The presence of fibrous adhesions on the pericardium indicated that inflammation had persisted for several weeks or more. Although hyaline arteriosclerosis, which can complicate diabetes, was specifically noted in the kidneys, spleen, and ovary at autopsy, it was probably present in small arteries throughout the body. Results of sterile postmortem cultures of blood, spleen, and lung specimens indicate that disseminated infection was not present at the end of this patient's course. Cultures of urine specimens, which might have identified the organism causing the pyelonephritis, were not performed because the patient's pyelonephritis was not suspected at the time the autopsy was begun. Information about the patient's possible osteomyelitis of the scapula and pelvis is also not included in the autopsy report. This deficit occurs because the usual autopsy procedure stresses examination of the chest and abdominal organs, and sometimes the brain and spinal cord, and generally does not involve dissection of other structures. These limitations are followed so that the appearance of the body can be preserved for a possible open-casket funeral. In light of the documented pericarditis, a possible reason for the patient's cardiorespiratory arrest was pericardial irritation leading to the development of an arrhythmia.

Septic Arthritis

A joint can become infected, producing infectious arthritis either by spread of infection from contiguous sources or by hematogenous dissemination of the organism. A septic joint can usually be easily treated with prompt therapy with appropriate antibiotics and surgical drainage of any abscesses if necessary. However, before the development of effective antibiotic therapy, septic arthritis was deeply dreaded because it was commonly complicated by dysfunction of the joint, osteomyelitis, and disseminated infection. The patient in this case followed a similar course since she did not receive adequate therapy until after her septic arthritis had been present for a considerable period. Although a very large variety of organisms are capable of causing septic arthritis, certain organisms are more often isolated in different age groups. *Staphylococcus aureus* and various streptococcal species are most commonly encountered in children; *Haemophilus influenzae, Neisseria gonorrhoeae,* and a variety of gram-negative bacilli are also found. In adults, *Neisseria gonorrhoeae* is the most common organism. *Staphylococcus aureus* and assorted streptococcal species are also frequently isolated.

Diabetic patients have often been noted to develop severe infections, including septic arthritis, more commonly than do most other patients. The basis for this vulnerability is still not fully understood, but appears to involve a combination of poor peripheral circulation leading to tissue vulnerability and decreased neutrophil function in the presence of high glucose levels. Infections in the extremities, particularly the legs, can occur after minor trauma. The resulting infections may be extremely difficult to control with antibiotics because of poor tissue perfusion leading to low antibiotic concentrations in the affected tissues. Severe urinary tract infections, such as this patient experienced, are also common, in part because any glucose in the urine can serve as a substrate for bacterial metabolism.

Questions

1. What chronic conditions did this patient have? How did her knee problems develop and progress? What might you do to improve this patient's willingness to accept medical care in a responsible manner?
2. What are the signs and symptoms related to this patient's knee disease? What is the differential diagnosis of her knee problems? Which findings tend to support or exclude each possible diagnosis? How is this patient's systemic disease related to her knee disease? How was her knee disease treated?
3. Discuss this patient's hospital course. How did each of her problems tend to predispose her to further complications? Which organ systems were eventually involved? What was found at autopsy?

Selected Reading

Cierny G, Mader JT: Approach to adult osteomyelitis. Orthop Rev 16:259–270, 1987.
DiMario U, Pugliese G: Diabetic complications: is there a way out of the labyrinth? J Diabetic Complications 2:163–166, 1988.
Klein RS: Joint infection, with consideration of underlying disease and sources of bacteremia in hematogenous infection. Clin Geriatr Med 4:375–394, 1988.
Leslie CA, Sapico FL, Bessman AN: Infections in the diabetic host. Compr Ther 15:23–32, 1989.

35 PROSTATIC ADENOCARCINOMA

Key Words | prostate cancer, metastatic disease, pneumonia

CASE

The patient was a 64-year-old man with a history of well-differentiated prostatic carcinoma diagnosed during a routine examination four years before. The patient had been on estrogen therapy since that time.[1] After metastatic cancer was diagnosed three years later, he underwent bilateral orchiectomy and irradiation of the spine, pelvis, and abdominal wall.[2] He was readmitted for pain relief four years after the initial diagnosis of prostatic carcinoma. He complained primarily of pain in the lumbrosacral spinal area, which was believed to be due to metastatic bone disease.[3]

The patient presented as a thin, cachectic man in no apparent distress. Physical examination revealed bilateral gynecomastia and a palpable tumor in the anterior pelvis. The prostate was firm and enlarged. Laboratory data were significant for a low hematocrit of 24% (normal, 40 to 52%) and a slight elevation in liver enzymes. The acid phosphatase was within normal limits. A chest radiograph taken at admission revealed prominent pulmonary vascular markings, and an electrocardiogram showed sinus tachycardia with a right bundle branch block. Bone scan showed multiple areas of increased uptake involving the ribs, spine, extremities, and skull (Fig. 35-1). The clinical impression was adenocarcinoma of the prostate with metastases. The patient also had chronic obstructive pulmonary disease.[4]

On admission, intravenous estrogen therapy

DISCUSSION

1. Both benign prostatic hypertrophy and prostatic carcinoma are often diagnosed when rectal examination reveals an enlarged prostate. The prostate is typically smooth in benign prostatic hypertrophy and nodular in prostatic carcinoma. These distinctions reflect only a general tendency, and the diagnosis must be confirmed by biopsy. High estrogen levels can suppress gonadotropin secretion by the pituitary and can consequently decrease testosterone production.

2. The patient's bilateral orchiectomy was intended to stop testosterone secretion. Unfortunately, although prostatic carcinoma may respond to estrogens, it is not responsive to most chemotherapeutic agents. Local radiation therapy may be helpful in prolonging the patient's life and controlling complications such as bone pain. It does not usually offer the possibility of a cure unless the cancer has not yet metastasized.

3. Relief of pain related to terminal cancer can be a substantial problem. Tumor involving bone, particularly in the vertebral column, can produce notoriously severe pain.

4. Cancer often produces cachexia, or extreme weight loss, by mechanisms that are still poorly understood. The patient's gynecomastia was the result of estrogen therapy. The presence of a palpable tumor suggests that a large tumor mass was present. The low hematocrit suggests that substantial tumor involvement of the bone marrow may have limited hematopoiesis. The slight elevation of liver enzymes indicated that hepatic metastases had developed. The pulmonary and cardio-

217

CASE

was started. The plan was that if a five-day course of intravenous estrogen did not relieve the pain, methadone treatment would be instituted. The patient continued to have significant pain, and methadone treatment was initiated two days after admission. The methadone dose was gradually increased in an attempt to control the pain and to produce a moderate level of comfort. Three days later the patient was noted to be nauseated and to have moderate dyspnea and some abdominal distension.[5] Arterial blood gas studies showed a respiratory acidosis, and oxygen administration via nasal cannula was begun. The next day, the patient was found to be hypoventilating. He was arousable and responsive. He continued to hypoventilate through the next day.[6] At that time, the pulmonary status had changed significantly to include rales throughout bilateral lung fields. The patient also exhibited jugular venous distension to the jaw. He was treated for pulmonary edema with diuretics and also bronchodilators, since he was in a positive fluid balance of approximately 3 L. His pain medicine was decreased to reverse his respiratory depression. Three days later, he was no longer short of breath, but he still complained of significant pain. The prognosis was discussed with the family. Both the patient and his family wanted primarily pain control and wished for no heroic measures to be taken.[7]

The patient continued to have significant bone pain, and intravenous morphine treatment was begun. The next day his temperature rose to 39.5°C (normal, 37.0°C), and blood, urine, and sputum specimens were obtained for culture. As per the family's wish, the intravenous morphine dose was increased even though respiratory depression developed. The next day, the 11th hospital day, the patient was noted to be pulseless and apneic and was pronounced dead. Culture of the urine specimen taken the day before his death revealed *Streptococcus faecalis* and *Proteus mirabilis*. Culture of the sputum specimen revealed light growth of *Proteus mirabilis*, moderate growth of *Streptococcus viridans*, and heavy growth of a coagulase-positive staphylococcus.[8]

At autopsy, nests and strands of poorly differentiated adenocarcinoma were seen in the pros-

DISCUSSION

vascular findings are not related to the patient's adenocarcinoma.

5. Estrogen therapy can rapidly control bone pain in many patients with disseminated prostatic cancer. Unfortunately this method was not successful in this patient. One of the complications of therapy with narcotics is respiratory depression. Respiratory depression can cause hypoxic damage to tissues. Also, a patient who is not breathing deeply, for whatever reason, has a markedly increased susceptibility to pneumonia.

6. The fact that the patient was arousable and responsive indicates that his condition was relatively stable despite the respiratory depression.

7. Rales and jugular venous distension suggest developing congestive heart failure with pulmonary edema. The patient's renal function may also have been impaired since he was in positive fluid balance. Potentially life-threatening decisions such as the decision to continue narcotic therapy should be made jointly. It is desirable that the physician, patient, and family

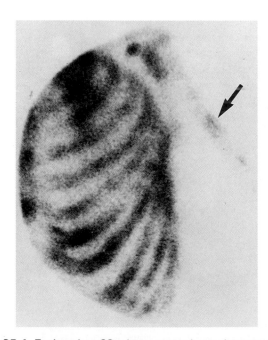

Fig. 35-1. Technetium 99m bone scan shows increased uptake in the left humerus *(arrow)*, suggestive of metastatic bone disease. Other metastatic sites were observed throughout the patient's skeleton.

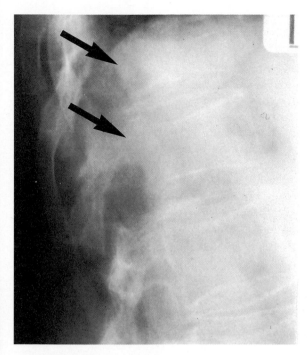

Fig. 35-2. Cancer involving vertebrae. The spinous processes of two vertebrae have been partially destroyed by cancer *(arrows)*.

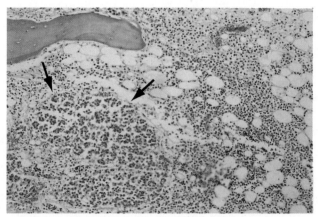

Fig. 35-3. Prostatic cancer involving bone marrow (low power photomicrograph, hematoxylin and eosin). The normal bone marrow has been partially replaced by nodules of prostatic adenocarcinoma *(arrows)*. In this field, the tumor appears to be forming glandlike structures.

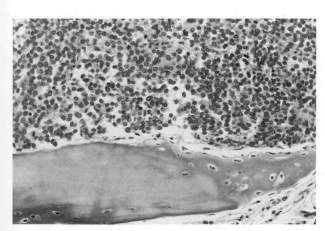

Fig. 35-4. Prostatic carcinoma involving bone (high power photomicrograph, hematoxylin and eosin). This higher power photomicrograph is taken from a different area of bone marrow than that shown in Fig. 35-3. The gland-forming ability of the tumor *(above)* in this field is less apparent than in Fig. 35-3.

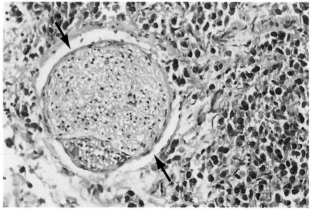

Fig. 35-5. Perineural tumor involvement (high power photomicrograph, hematoxylin and eosin). One mechanism of tumor spread in prostatic cancer is by invasion of perineural lymphatics. A small nerve *(arrows)* can be seen; adjacent surrounding tissues *(right)* show extensive tumor invasion. The severe pain associated with disseminated carcinoma can be due to compression of nerves as well as to direct involvement of the nerves with tumor.

CASE

tate. There was widespread metastasis of tumor to lung, bone, and lymph nodes (Figs. 35-2 to 35-5). The tumor was noted to have spread lymphatogenously along the pulmonary arteries, with resultant diffuse involvement of the lungs. There were sheets of tumor cells replacing the normal marrow elements. The patient had had bone pain, lymphadenopathy, and extramedullary hematopoiesis, all of which were consistent with myelophthisic anemia. Scattered diffusely throughout the lungs was a purulent exudate that filled the bronchi and flooded the alveoli. The cause of death was considered to be acute bronchopneumonia in a patient with widely metastatic prostatic adenocarcinoma.[9]

DISCUSSION

reach a consensus about what should be done. Any discussions with the family should be carefully documented in the medical record for both medical and legal reasons.

8. Not all physicians would agree to increase the morphine dose in a terminally ill patient with respiratory depression, since the resulting respiratory depression may be the proximate cause of the patient's death. This ethical dilemma may be resolved differently by different physicians. Urinary tract infection is common in patients with prostatic cancer, partly because the tumor may cause urinary retention and partly because tumor involvement of the bladder may impair normal physiological defenses.

9. The patient's cancer metastasized widely by an apparently predominantly lymphatic route. Myelophthisic anemia is caused by replacement of bone marrow by tumor or other tissue. The pneumonia suspected by the premortem sputum cultures was confirmed by the autopsy findings.

Prostate Cancer

Prostatic carcinoma is the second most common cancer in men, but only approximately one-third of cases recognized at autopsy were diagnosed clinically. Prostate carcinoma may follow an indolent course or behave aggressively. Most of the cancers are adenocarcinomas that tend to develop in peripheral prostatic acini. A few are transitional cell or squamous cell carcinomas. The tumors are frequently multifocal. This suggests that the pathogenesis of the tumor involves a field effect in which a predisposition to the development of cancer affects many cells. The tumors are typically diagnosed during digital rectal examination, when a hard and nodular prostate is palpated. Biopsy is required to confirm the diagnosis since fibrous areas in benign prostatic hypertrophy may produce similar findings on rectal examination.

Therapies vary depending on the size of the tumor and the degree to which it has metastasized. In the absence of widespread metastasis, either simple prostatec-

tomy or radical prostatectomy, including removal of the prostate and seminal vesicles, may be appropriate. External beam radiation therapy can be used as a primary treatment in localized prostatic carcinoma and for palliation of bone pain due to metastasis. Seeds of ^{125}I can also be implanted as a radiation source if a well-defined, small tumor mass is present. The growth of the normal prostate and many prostatic carcinomas requires androgen. Androgen deprivation can be accomplished by a variety of techniques including removal of testes and adrenal glands; inhibition of pituitary production of gonadotropin by hypophysectomy; and treatment with estrogens or luteinizing hormone-releasing analogs. Aminoglutethimide can inhibit androgen synthesis by the testes and adrenal glands. Cyproterone and flutamide can block the binding of androgen to its receptors. Unfortunately, although androgen deprivation is in widespread use, it has not been shown to improve survival. It can, however, relieve bone pain due to metastases in many patients. Other chemotherapeutic strategies have not been very successful.

Questions

1. How was this patient's prostatic carcinoma diagnosed? What types of treatment were used to control his prostatic carcinoma? What was their rationale? What tissues were known to be involved by his tumor at the time of his final admission?
2. What were the patient's presenting complaints at his final admission? What did physical examination and laboratory studies show at that time? What methods were used to treat his pain? What factors influenced the decisions about how much medication he would receive for pain therapy?
3. What happened to this patient's respiratory status during his admission? How did he die? What evidence before the patient's death suggested that he had an infection? What evidence of infection was found at autopsy? Describe the extent of the patient's metastases as observed at autopsy.

Selected Reading

Freiha FS, Bayshaw MA, Torti FM: Carcinoma of the prostate: pathology, staging, and treatment. Curr Probl Cancer 12:329–411, 1988.

Meares EM: Urinary tract infections in the male patient. Urology 32:19–20, 1988.

Payne R, Foley KM: Cancer pain. Med Clin N Am 71:153–348, 1987.

36 MENINGOCOCCEMIAL SEPSIS WITH WATERHOUSE-FRIDERICHSEN SYNDROME

Key Words

meningococci, sepsis, Waterhouse-Friderichsen syndrome

CASE

A 20-year-old man presented to the emergency room after one day of malaise, nausea, and vomiting that progressed to myalgias, arthralgias, and rash. Vital signs included blood pressure of 60 mmHg systolic (normal, 100 to 140/60 to 90 mmHg), a pulse of 150/min (normal, 60 to 100/min), a respiratory rate of 50/min (normal, 6 to 20/min), and a temperature of 38°C (normal, 37°C). Administration of 5 L of intravenous fluid raised his blood pressure to greater than 100 mmHg systolic. However, he then developed marked respiratory distress, and results of a physical examination were consistent with pulmonary edema.[1] He was immediately treated with morphine sulfate and with intravenous furosemide. Only 100 ml of urine was produced. He was taken to the medical intensive care unit, where he was given two ampules of naloxone. He continued to have respiratory distress combined with acidosis and consequently was intubated.[2]

Physical examination in the medical intensive care unit revealed a blood pressure of 95/62

DISCUSSION

1. This patient's rapidly developing course suggests that he was seriously ill. The conjunction of fever, hypotension, tachycardia, and tachypnea strongly suggests septic shock. Organisms frequently isolated from the bloodstream in septic shock include *Escherichia coli, Klebsiella, Enterobacter, Proteus, Pseudomonas, Serratia,* and *Neisseria meningitidis*. The fluid losses to interstitial tissue in septic shock can be very large. Restoration of blood volume is critical to survival. Unfortunately, fluid loss from the vascular space often continues; in this case it led to the development of pulmonary edema.

2. The diuretic furosemide was administered to try to reverse the pulmonary edema. The failure of the diuretic to increase urine output indicates that the patient had developed acute renal failure, probably due to acute tubular necrosis secondary to shock. Despite his severe discomfort, the administration of morphine was a mistake because it can cause respiratory depression. Naloxone reverses the effect of morphine. Respiratory acidosis can be produced by carbon dioxide retention in a hypoventilating patient.

223

CASE

mmHg, a pulse of 132/min, a respiratory rate of 30/min, and a temperature of 38°C. Marked acrocyanosis of the hands and feet was present. He also had nonblanching, nonpalpable purpura distributed diffusely over the arms, legs, and trunk.[3] Examination of the head was remarkable for conjunctival petechiae. The nose and throat were unremarkable. There was no lymphadenopathy, and only mild neck rigidity. Examination of the lungs revealed scattered rhonchi.[4]

Laboratory data taken after the transfusions in the emergency room revealed sodium of 134 mEq/L (normal, 137 to 145 mEq/L), chloride of 94 mEq/L (normal, 94 to 107 mEq/L), potassium of 2.9 mEq/L (normal, 3.6 to 5.0 mEq/L), and bicarbonate of 18 mEq/L (normal, 24 to 30 mEq/L). Blood urea nitrogen was 26 mg/100 ml (normal, 6 to 20 mg/100 ml), and creatinine was 4.8 mg/100 ml (normal, 0.5 to 1.4 mg/100 ml).[5] A peripheral white blood cell count was 14,200/mm³ (normal, 4,500 to 11,000/mm³) with 47% mature neutrophils (normal, 40 to 70%) and 36% band forms (normal, 0 to 5%). Platelet counts were

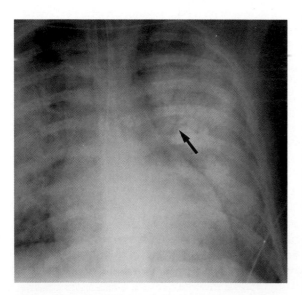

Fig. 36-1. Radiograph of the chest shows diffuse alveolar infiltration with air bronchograms *(arrow)*. These changes were interpreted as being consistent with severe pulmonary edema.

DISCUSSION

Metabolic acidosis can accompany sepsis. More severe acidosis is observed when both respiratory and metabolic acidosis are present, since physiologic compensatory mechanisms are impaired.

3. Before shock develops fully, generalized vasoconstriction is present that helps to improve venous return. The patient's extremities were consequently cold and cyanotic (acrocyanosis). As hypotension develops, compensatory tachypnea and tachycardia also develop. Severe hemorrhage within the skin causes rapidly enlarging petechiae and purpuric lesions that may cover the entire body. The clinical pattern is suggestive of fulminant meningococcemia, although other diseases, including Rocky Mountain spotted fever, can produce a similar picture.

4. Neck rigidity was checked in this patient as a test for possible meningitis. The presence of conjunctival petechiae confirmed that the hemorrhage was not limited to the skin.

5. Low or low normal values for many electrolytes indicate that the transfusion may have restored slightly more than the necessary fluids, with resulting mild hemodilution. High blood urea nitrogen and creatinine levels confirm developing renal failure. Given that the patient presumably had normal levels several days earlier, these values are quite high.

6. Leukocytosis, and in particular increased immature forms, may indicate infection. More slowly developing signs such as lymphadenopathy are usually not present in fulminant meningococcemia. The patient is initially alert, but if he lives long enough, coma may develop. Fever, arthralgia, and muscle pain are common. Platelet counts are decreased secondary to consumption in disseminated intravascular coagulation.

7. This patient's history and physical examination showed many of the classic features of fulminant meningococcemia, also known as the Waterhouse-Friderichsen syndrome. Most patients either are normal or have mild cold symptoms before developing meningococcemia. Meningococci are most often harbored asymptomatically in the nasopharynx. However, they may cause either a serious form of meningitis, which usually occurs in children, or a life-threatening bacteremia, which usually occurs in young adults. Previous vaccination against appropriate strains may prevent development of meningococ-

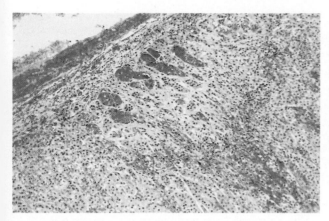

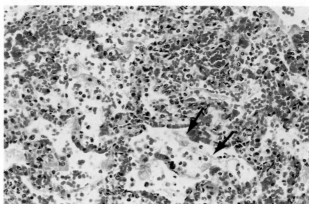

Fig. 36-2. Adrenal hemorrhage (low power photomicrograph, hematoxylin and eosin). The adrenal cortex is particularly vulnerable to decreased perfusion and may develop diffuse hemorrhage, such as illustrated in this field, when shock occurs.

Fig. 36-3. Diffuse alveolar damage (high power photomicrograph, hematoxylin and eosin). This lung, which has been damaged by shock, has sustained diffuse damage to the capillary bed, leading to alveolar hemorrhage. Desquamated alveolar pneumocytes *(arrows)* can also be seen in the alveoli. When decreased perfusion to the lung is generalized, as occurs in shock, the damage to the lung is widespread and can significantly limit the ability to oxygenate blood.

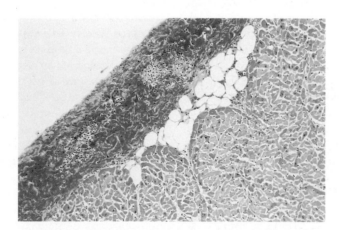

Fig. 36-4. Pericardial hemorrhage (low power photomicrograph, hematoxylin and eosin). Significant pericardial hemorrhage *(upper left)* has also occurred in this patient, by mechanisms similar to the adrenal and alveolar hemorrhage illustrated in previous figures. The cardiac muscle *(lower right)* shows inhomogeneous staining of muscle fibers, suggesting that damage to muscle fibers has also occurred.

CASE

96,000/mm^3 (normal, 150,000 to 450,000/mm^3).[6] Early results of the blood smear examination revealed gram-negative diplococci in neutrophils. A cerebrospinal fluid sample contained 2,000 neutrophils per mm^3 and what was thought to be gram-negative diplococci in the neutrophils.[7] The patient denied any history of infectious disease, penile discharges, or homosexuality. Culture of one blood specimen grew *Neisseria meningitidis*. The prothrombin time and partial thromboblastin time were both markedly prolonged. A chest radiograph showed early reticular fluffy infiltrates. Examination of a urine specimen revealed hematuria (1+), proteinuria (4+), many granular casts, and rare leukocytes and erythrocytes.[8]

The impression on admission was probable sepsis, with meningococcemia a likely candidate. Disseminated intravascular coagulation was present. Renal failure was thought to be due to acute tubular necrosis. The patient was treated with fluids and the intravenous antibiotics chloramphenicol and vancomycin.[9] He initially appeared stable during the one day of hospitalization. That night, he developed a severe hypoxia, which was not responsive to increased oxygen concentration or ventilatory pressures. A chest radiograph showed severe pulmonary edema (Fig. 36-1). He also developed severe lactic acidosis. It appeared as though he had an arteriovenous shunting phenomenon through the lungs. Resuscitative efforts failed, and he died.[10]

Autopsy revealed evidence of shock, including diffuse alveolar damage, acute tubular necrosis of the kidneys, and focal ischemic necrosis of the heart (Figs. 36-2 to 36-4). Subacute leptomeningitis was also present. All of the features of classic Waterhouse-Friderichsen syndrome were present. These include shock, sepsis, disseminated intravascular coagulation, and marked hemorrhagic necrosis of both adrenal glands. This syndrome is most often associated with meningococcemial sepsis, but is occasionally seen with other infective organisms.[11]

DISCUSSION

cal infections. The diagnosis is typically confirmed by finding intracellular gram-negative diplococci which are confirmed on culture to be *Neisseria meningitis* (meningococci). In this patient, the probable presence of meningococci in cerebrospinal fluid indicates that the bacteria were present in the central nervous system even though they had not caused clinical meningitis. The onset of fulminant meningococcemia is usually abrupt, and many patients become very ill within a few hours.

8. The patient's sexual history was elicited to rule against gonorrhea, which is caused by another gram-negative intracellular diplococcus, and exotic infections associated with acquired immune deficiency syndrome (AIDS). The positive blood culture confirmed the diagnosis of systemic meningococcemia. Additional evidence of the coagulation disturbance was indicated by the prolonged prothrombin and partial thromboplastin times. The pulmonary infiltrates may have been due to the combination of pulmonary edema and alveolar hemorrhage. Adult respiratory distress syndrome was probably developing. The urine studies gave findings typical of acute tubular necrosis.

9. Rapid treatment with appropriate antibiotics and control of shock and its manifestations form the basis of therapeutic strategy in fulminant meningococcemia. Massive doses of adrenal cortical steroids, although not used in this case, may also be helpful. Unfortunately, fulminant meningococcemia has a high mortality rate, so even appropriate and prompt therapy, as this patient received, is not always successful. Since the mortality rate is so high, people who have had contact with the patient (medical staff, family, and school or work contacts) should be given prophylactic antibiotic therapy.

10. Lactic acidosis is due to tissue destruction produced by ischemia, hypotension, and disseminated intravascular coagulation. Severe hypoxia and pulmonary vascular congestion are typical of adult respiratory distress syndrome. Results of blood gas studies apparently consistent with an arteriovenous shunting phenomenon were actually due to perfusion of alveoli that were not being ventilated because they were filled with edema and hemorrhage.

11. Subacute leptomeningitis indicated meningeal infec-

tion. Clinical meningitis characteristically takes somewhat longer to develop than fulminant meningococcemia, and consequently is usually seen only in patients who do not develop bacteremia with the accompanying pattern of fulminant meningococcemia. The adrenal glands are particularly vulnerable to damage by hypotension, which causes hemorrhagic necrosis. This damage can produce irreversible adrenal failure, requiring replacement therapy in patients who survive.

Shock

A sustained, pronounced decrease in perfusion will damage all body tissues and lead rapidly to death. The body has some ability to compensate for milder states of shock, and this ability to compensate may often be augmented by appropriate therapy. In such cases, some organs are much more vulnerable than others to serious damage by shock. Renal proximal tubule cells are particularly vulnerable to ischemia; acute tubular necrosis causes acute renal failure. The heart characteristically shows focal areas of necrosis and hemorrhage after severe shock. Shock damage to the lungs causes adult respiratory distress syndrome, characterized by necrosis of the alveolar epithelium and endothelial cells, microthrombi, interstitial edema, and acute inflammatory cells. The mucosa of the large and small bowel is also vulnerable to ischemic necrosis. The development of septicemia may be related to interruption of the barrier function of the intestinal mucosa. Duodenal ulcer and rupture of the esophagus can also occur. The spleen may show congestion and hyperplasia. The liver may show centrilobular hemorrhagic necrosis. Ischemic damage to the pancreas releases activated catalytic enzymes and causes acute pancreatitis. Patients suffering from shock are also very vulnerable to infection. Brain lesions are rare, but hemorrhage and necrosis may occur in the so-called "watershed zone" between the terminal distributions of major arteries. The adrenal glands may exhibit significant hemorrhage and necrosis, as is seen in the Waterhouse-Friderichsen syndrome. If the patient survives the shock, clinical adrenal failure may be present and require lifelong replacement therapy with glucocorticoids and mineralocorticoids.

Questions

1. What were this patient's presenting complaints? Which features of his presentation suggested that he was dangerously ill? How was he initially treated? What respiratory problem did he develop? Why was the morphine treatment a mistake?
2. Which features of this patient's presentation suggested meningococcemial sepsis? What other diseases should have been included in the differential diagnosis? Discuss the patient's laboratory studies. Why was a low platelet count a cause for concern?
3. Which organ systems are particularly vulnerable to shock? What clinical evidence of organ damage did this patient manifest? What is the Waterhouse-Friderichsen syndrome? Why is it dangerous? Relate the findings at autopsy to this patient's clinical course.

Selected Reading

Tunkel AR, Wispelway B, Scheld WM: Bacterial meningitis: recent advances in pathophysiology and treatment. Ann Intern Med 112:610–623, 1990.

Wall RA: The chemoprophylaxis of meningococcal infection. J Antimicrob Chemother 21:698–700, 1988.

Wong VK, Agee B, Kim KS, Wright HT: Meningococcal infections. West J Med 150:68–73, 1989.

37 HASHIMOTO'S THYROIDITIS

Key Words | thyroid mass, Hashimoto's thyroiditis, stroke, meningitis

CASE

A 57-year-old woman was admitted for evaluation of right arm and right leg weakness, which was subsequently diagnosed as having been due to a stroke. Physical examination revealed a massive, diffusely enlarged thyroid gland, with the right lobe more involved than the left. There was no regional or more distal lymphadenopathy.[1] Approximately two months earlier she had noted a "bump" on her neck, but she had thought that the mass was "swollen glands" and had consequently not sought medical attention. She could "feel the bump" when she stretched her neck or lifted her arms above her head, but otherwise the mass was not noticeable to her. She denied heat or cold intolerance, change in voice, palpitations, and breathing difficulties.[2] She had no history of neck irradiation. Her family history was positive for thyroidectomy in her mother and for nodules with thyroid replacement in two nieces. Thyroid studies showed normal triiodothyronine (T3), T3 resin uptake, and thyroxine (T4). Thyroid-stimulating hormone (TSH) was 21 μU/ml (normal, <6 μU/ml). Immunologic studies were strongly positive for anti-thyroid microsomal antibodies.[3]

In addition to her thyroid nodule and her stroke, several other medical problems were evident at admission. She had an unexplained mild anemia and mild leukopenia. She had also had bacterial meningitis following a myelogram performed during evaluation of her stroke. Following this meningitis, repeated spinal taps showed normal lymphocytes in the cerebrospinal fluid.[4]

DISCUSSION

1. One of the reasons for performing a careful physical examination on any patient during admission is that unsuspected medical problems, unrelated to the patient's presenting complaints, may be identified. Causes of thyroid masses can be classed as those producing diffuse thyroid enlargement, those producing multinodularity, and those producing a solitary thyroid nodule. Diffuse thyroid enlargement can be caused by, among others, Graves' disease, diffuse colloid goiter, and thyroiditis.

2. It is somewhat surprising that this patient's large neck mass had not produced more symptoms. Heat intolerance would have suggested hyperthyroidism; cold intolerance would have suggested hypothyroidism. Hyperthyroidism can also increase the heart rate, which can be experienced by patients as palpitations. Compression of the trachea by a mass can produce breathing difficulties. Change in the voice can be produced either by direct pressure on the vocal cords or by compression of the nerve supply to the vocal cords, particularly the recurrent laryngeal nerve that runs near the thyroid gland.

3. Neck irradiation is associated with increased incidence of thyroid cancer. Head and neck irradiation was formerly a common treatment for recurrent childhood infections. The family history of thyroid disease is consistent with many thyroid diseases. T3 and T4 are the active thyroid hormones. T3 resin uptake is a measure of the capacity of serum proteins to bind additional thyroid hormone. TSH is produced by the pituitary and acts on the thyroid gland to stimulate thyroid growth and to increase the release of T3 and T4.

CASE

Although thyroiditis was the most strongly suspected diagnosis of her thyroid mass, lymphoma, particularly a primary thyroid lymphoma, was also suspected since it might account for her anemia, leukopenia, and vulnerability to meningitis. A core biopsy of the thyroid mass was read as consistent with chronic lymphocytic thyroiditis, but neither her clinical history nor the needle biopsy was able to definitely distinguish between primary thyroid lymphoma and Hashimoto's thyroiditis. It was decided that she would require an open tissue biopsy for diagnosis. This biopsy was deferred while a trial administration of synthetic thyroid hormone was used to "rest" the remaining thyroid tissue.[5]

Six months later, the patient was admitted for same-day surgery for thyroidectomy. Findings at surgery showed a diffusely indurated thyroid, which was very hard and could not be safely freed from surrounding tissue. The trachea was decompressed, and a large segment of the thyroid was sent for histological study. Postoperatively, the patient did well and was discharged home on the second postoperative day, without complications.[6]

Extensive immunohistochemical evaluation of the biopsy was performed by using immunoperoxidase techniques for a wide variety of immunoglobulins and B- and T-cell markers. These studies showed that the lymphoid cell population was polyclonal, which was considered to be more consistent with a reactive than a neoplastic proliferation of lymphoid elements in the thyroid (Figs. 37-1 to 37-3). Consequently, a diagnosis of Hashimoto's thyroiditis was made.[7]

DISCUSSION

The patient's normal T3, T3 resin uptake, and T4 results mean that she was euthyroid, which was consistent with her clinically observed absence of symptoms of hypo- or hyperthyroidism. However, the elevation of the TSH level suggests that even though she was euthyroid, her thyroid gland was requiring strong stimulation to maintain this state. The presence of anti-thyroid antibodies suggests that the patient's thyroid gland may be enlarged as a result of autoimmune disease.

4. Procedures such as spinal tap or myelogram potentially introduce small numbers of bacteria into the cerebrospinal fluid even when a sterile technique is used. Clinically significant meningitis following such procedures is uncommon and suggests that some other pathological process may have predisposed the patient to infection. Normal cerebrospinal fluid contains only a very few white blood cells. The patient's mild anemia, mild leukopenia, and vulnerability to meningitis may simply have been coincidental phenomena whose explanation will never be fully identified. However, their simultaneous occurrence also suggests that they are a cluster of clinical findings occurring in response to a single underlying pathological process.

5. In both Hashimoto's thyroiditis and lymphoma involving the thyroid gland, the thyroid tissue can be diffusely replaced by proliferating lymphoid elements. In lymphoma, there is a tumorous proliferation of the lymphoid elements. In Hashimoto's thyroiditis, the lymphocytes are reactive lymphocytes, which produce antibodies directed against thyroid antigens. These thyroid antigens are often thyroid microsomal (endoplasmic reticulum) elements and TSH receptors, but may also be thyroglobulin, other colloid proteins, or follicular cell membranes. In both thyroiditis and lymphoma involving the thyroid, the patient may eventually become hypothyroid as the amount of functioning thyroid tissue diminishes. It has been observed that some recovery of thyroid function sometimes occurs in thyroiditis if TSH levels drop in response to exogenously administered thyroid hormone.

6. The major risks of thyroid surgery are damage to the many important nerves and vessels of the neck or to the parathyroid glands. These risks were increased in this patient by the consistency of the tumor. Its hardness was related to replacement of normal thyroid fol-

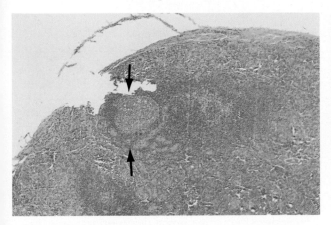

Fig. 37-1. Hashimoto's thyroiditis (low power photomicrograph, hematoxylin and eosin). The normal follicular architecture of this thyroid gland has been so completely disrupted by thyroiditis that the tissue is difficult to recognize as thyroid. A lymphoid germinal center *(arrows)* can be recognized.

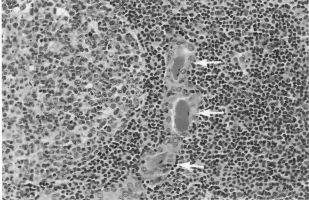

Fig. 37-2. Hashimoto's thyroiditis, detail of Fig. 37-1 (high power photomicrograph, hematoxylin and eosin). To the left is an enlarged view of the maturing B cells in the lymphoid germinal center marked by the arrow in Fig. 37-1. In the center of the field are three thyroid follicular remnants *(arrows)* that are still producing small quantities of colloid. To the right is a dense infiltration of mature lymphocytes. These lymphocytes are associated with the autoimmune destruction of the thyroid gland in Hashimoto's disease.

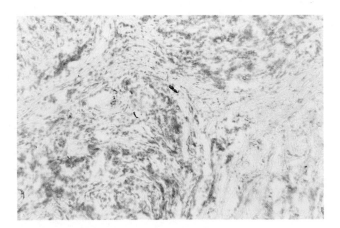

Fig. 37-3. Hashimoto's thyroiditis (high power photomicrograph, immunological stain for B cells). Immunological staining for B-cell markers in this patient shows a polyclonal population in which some cells stain for B-cell markers (brownish cells) while others do not (bluish cells). Staining for other cell markers produced qualitatively similar results. These results indicate that the lymphocytic proliferation is a reactive, polyclonal proliferation, rather than a neoplastic, monoclonal proliferation such as would be produced by lymphoma.

DISCUSSION

licles by masses of lymphocytes and scar tissue. For this patient, it was decided to do only enough dissection to relieve the compression of the trachea by the mass, rather than to attempt complete removal of the thyroid.

7. Immunohistochemical techniques have markedly improved the ability to accurately diagnose a variety of pathological processes, particularly tumors and processes involving the immune system. The immunoperoxidase technique is based on chemically binding the enzyme peroxidase to a commercially available antibody directed against a particular antigen of interest. The antigen may be a normal or abnormal tissue constituent, or it may itself be an antibody. The coupled peroxidase-antibody molecules will then bind to any of the antigen present in the tissue. When the tissue sections are later exposed to appropriate reagents, the peroxidase part of the complex produces a visible dark-brown or black precipitate. For this patient, the rationale for using immunoperoxidase techniques directed against a variety of antigens was that a lymphoma would be expected to contain a population of cells with uniform or near-uniform surface antigens, whereas a reactive leukocytosis would be expected to contain a mixture of lymphocytes expressing a variety of antigens. Since the patient's disease proved to be Hashimoto's thyroiditis rather than lymphoma, the prognosis is good. She will probably continue to require thyroid hormone supplementation and may need a second decompressive surgery at some later date if her thyroiditis continues to involve adjacent structures.

Hashimoto's Thyroiditis

Hashimoto's thyroiditis is a thyroid condition characterized by replacement of thyroid follicles by lymphoid elements. Although the complete cause and progression have not been elucidated, Hashimoto's thyroiditis appears to be an autoimmune disease in which autoantibodies can be directed against a variety of normal thyroid antigens. Frequently demonstrated antibodies include those directed against thyroid microsomal fractions and those directed against TSH receptors. Antibodies are also sometimes found that are directed against other thyroid proteins, including thyroglobulin, other colloid proteins, and follicular cell membrane proteins.

In contrast to the autoantibodies directed against TSH receptors present in Graves' disease, the autoantibodies in Hashimoto's thyroiditis do not cause hypersecretion of thyroid hormones. They do, however, stimulate thyroid growth, leading to the formation of an enlarged, hard thyroid gland. Microscopically, the thyroid tissue is almost completely replaced by sheets of lymphocytes containing germinal centers. The few remaining follicles are characteristically degenerated, and the follicular epithelium is metaplastic.

Hashimoto's thyroiditis characteristically occurs in perimenopausal women. Clinical symptoms are related to the size and location of the thyroid mass, which is often quite large, and are also related to the hypothyroidism that may eventually develop.

Questions

1. How did this patient present? What were her medical problems? Were they related?
2. What types of pathological process can produce a neck mass? Describe this patient's symptoms related to her neck mass. What other symptoms might she have experienced?
3. What diagnoses were considered for the patient's thyroid mass? Why was each diagnosis considered? How was the diagnosis made? What was found at surgery?

Selected Reading

Charreire J: Immune mechanisms in autoimmune thyroiditis. Adv Immunol 46:263–334, 1987.

De Baers MH: Autoimmune endocrine diseases. Year Immunol 4:264–275, 1989.

Hay ID, Klee GG: Thyroid dysfunction. Endocrinol Metab Clin N Am 17:473–509, 1988.

INDEX

Note: Numbers followed by an f indicate figures.